CONQUER EMOTIONAL EATING

OVERCOME NEGATIVE THOUGHTS AND SELF-SABOTAGE. TAKE CONTROL OF YOUR BODY AND YOUR LIFE TODAY.

ELLA RENÉE

CONTENTS

Introduction   5

1. Are You Eating Your Emotions?   13
2. The Problem with Weight Loss   31
3. Lead Your Thoughts   47
4. Evade Your Triggers   67
5. Tune in to Your Emotions   89
6. Give in to Your Real Needs   115
7. Observe and Obey Your True Hunger   133
8. Practical Ways to Support Healthy Eating   151

Conclusion   175
Bibliography   179

INTRODUCTION

> "*Food can distract you from your pain. But food cannot take away your pain. In fact, overeating the wrong foods can create more pain.*"

> — KAREN SALMANSOHN

Eating your emotions is easy comedy material for Hollywood. Just ask Elle Woods, who got dumped by her boyfriend and went on a steep downward spiral, with a box of chocolates seemingly as her only friend. It's great for a few laughs until the next joke comes up and the previous scene is completely erased from your mind. Meanwhile, in real life, there's no queue of jokes to distract you from a garbage bin filled with empty ice cream tubs and a tower of grease-stained pizza boxes on your kitchen counter. You're horrified at the sight, but it doesn't immediately register in your brain that these are all the collateral damage of your grief, pain, guilt, self-loathing, and a host of other negative emotions fighting for space inside you.

Emotional eating sounds like a great reason for a fun cheat day when you can let yourself go and not worry about calories, clogged arteries, or a smashed piggy bank to pay for all those Cheetos. You need it. You deserve it. You have all those hungry feelings to feed. That's all that matters. Not your zero bank balance. Not your nasty boss. Not your ailing significant other.

Stuffing yourself with food because you're upset about the cast turnover in *Grey's Anatomy* isn't about satisfying a physical hunger. It has absolutely nothing to do with the natural cravings of your body but everything to do with your unnatural reaction to the things going on inside and around you. A negative emotion is burning a hole in your innermost being and you're casting about for something—anything—to fill the void. And so, you set your sights on food, which literally packs the hollow chambers of your tummy. As the whole rotisserie chicken sits in your stomach, it tricks your mind into believing that all is finally well because the emptiness inside you has disappeared. Meanwhile, what's actually happening is that you're piling on the pounds that end up in your chin, upper arms, waist, hips, and thighs. When you see your reflection in the mirror, your chest suddenly constricts and you feel unbearable sadness that can only be washed away by two liters of your favorite soft drink. Before the month is over, you can no longer zip yourself up in the lovely party dress that cost you a kidney, so you reach for the fridge door to make yourself feel better and another vicious cycle begins.

If you're a woman determined to maintain the weight that's ideal for you (depending on your height, age, and other scientific/medical factors, of course, not what some social media influencer says), then you've just met one of your most ruthless enemies face-to-face: your emotions. According to a survey of 1,328 licensed psychologists, your emotions can make or break your weight goals. As the earlier tale shows, emotions can take you on a very wild, endless rollercoaster ride. No one else can put the brakes on it except you. It's no surprise then that 44 percent of the psych experts surveyed recommend knowing and controlling your actions and emotions to achieve success in your weight management. For as long as you don't have a handle on it, emotional eating, binge eating, or starvation can continue to dominate your life—even without your knowing it—and keep you away from your much-desired body weight. That knowledge and power over your emotions coupled with a set exercise regimen and the right eating habits and choices are the golden ticket to your ideal beach bod, mom bod, or simply healthy bod. It sounds simple enough except that in this age of instant gratification, FOMO (fear of missing out), and YOLO (you only live once), self-control seems to be the last thing you want to practice. However, the professional word and evidence is right here: mastery over your behaviors and emotions can help you lose or gain weight, whichever is your goal.

When your favorite Chinese resto is on speed-dial for a solo banquet after rough days at work or a whole drawer in your nightstand is full to the brim with chocolate bars, chewy toffees, and gummy bears for your "Netflix and chill" nights alone, that's you feeding your stress and loneliness. The foodstuff itself is not the problem; it's your emotions that prompt you to indulge in them even though you've already eaten and are quite full. It's a compulsion—like being on autopilot because that's what your mind remembers and what your body has been programmed to do. You might even attempt to go to the other extreme and starve yourself. Neither the gluttony nor the deprivation makes you feel good about yourself afterward. You only end up hating food and drowning in self-condemnation over the whole situation because none of it makes sense and it just seems to be getting worse every day. You're just about ready to give up on your weight goals and raise a white flag of surrender.

While it may feel like it from where you currently sit, it's not the end of the world. You're not under some eternal curse that can never be broken. There is a way out of your predicament and it begins with this: knowing that you have so many other options for coping with your emotions without involving food in the equation. That's the first benefit that you can derive from reading this book. You and I are going to work together on discovering better ways to deal with your emotions. To do that, we'll dig deep into your relationship with food and its connection to your emotions. Lastly and most importantly, this book will help you learn to love and take care of yourself. When you can do this, no amount of changing winds and tides in your life will make you want to go back to your former and unwanted weight status. To recap all that, reading and taking this book to heart can support you in:

- Learning new ways to manage your emotions without using food as a solution.
- Understanding the relationship between food and your emotions in order to break the unhealthy ties for your own good, and
- Loving and taking better care of yourself.

This book doesn't promise you a magic carpet ride—you might end up in dark corners of yourself that are uncomfortable to confront, but it does point the way toward you becoming the healthiest you could ever be. You're going to love and embrace the person you are, standing in front of a mirror, unafraid and unashamed. Your mind and heart will float light and carefree, unburdened by guilt and no longer slaves to compulsive behaviors. You'll find more exciting, productive, and meaningful ways of coping with personal crises away from and beyond easy food fixes. You're going to discover that there's more to you than what food has defined for years. You're going to put in the work and reward yourself with the life—and weight—that you've always wanted.

I don't take my role as your cheerleader lightly. I've also put in my own share of the work. For almost 20 years now, I've helped hundreds of women lose weight and achieve a healthy and well-balanced lifestyle. I'm here for each individual. As with each client, I see you. I hear you. I seek to know you. If you're yearning for a more permanent solution to your weight issues, then I'm here to say that there is one. The key is in recognizing that the real problem lies beyond the physical. Weight management begins with overcoming negative thoughts and self-sabotage. Once you can take care of the root, the rest of you can thrive.

While I may not be there for you physically right now, I hope this book fills the gap of my absence. I write this because I want to reach as many women—and men—as possible with my simple message: you can change your weight by changing the way you think. If your bodily heft bugs you and the weighing scale is a nemesis in your bathroom, then my proxy (this book) is on hand to encourage you that it doesn't have to be that way for you forever. You can take charge of your body and health. You are not meant to be obese/overweight until your very last breath. Once you learn that weight management is a mental exercise, you'll be able to hurdle many (mental) barriers along the way and make your weight management journey so much easier.

I'm meeting you right where you are now. I'm taking you as-is. Do you know how some people floss and brush and gargle thoroughly just before they go to their dentist for their regular cleaning? Well, you don't have to do that kind of nonsense with me. Come as you are and let's make good things happen for you, wherever your starting point is.

1

ARE YOU EATING YOUR EMOTIONS?

Whenever I have a chance to rewatch some of my favorite movies from childhood, I'm always amazed at how kids back then seemed to be in perpetual motion—biking, hiking, climbing, running, etc. They stopped just long enough to empty their plates for a meal or a snack before taking off again for the next adventure, the next clue, the next discovery. They rushed home only when the streetlights came on and supper was laid out on the dining table. From the sweaty smiles on their faces, you couldn't mistake it to be anything but a great day for them. It was my good fortune to have had the same childhood, too.

I think about that fun and carefree life and notice something important: as children, my friends and I ate food to replenish our expended energies and sustain the vitality of our bodies. We didn't eat because we had nothing else to do or were craving a particular taste or needed to keep our mouths as busy as our hands as we played video games. In other words, eating was—and still is—essential but not the centerpiece of our lives.

These days, it's hard not to have food front and center of your every waking moment. Just stroll into any of the gargantuan supermarket chains and see aisle upon aisle of breads, cereals, chips, cheeses, sauces, etc. The choices are so vast; they're mind-boggling. Restaurants, food trucks, and kiosks offer a cornucopia of international cuisine as you drive by on your way to an appointment. I bet you even have at least one app or one number on your phone for food delivery. When you switch to any of your social media accounts, it's very likely that there'll be more posts about food and eating than the alarming state of global climate change.

With food practically in your face at every turn, it's very clear that this society's views of and values about food and eating are very different from your parents' … and even grandparents'. Food is not just there as sustenance and energy-giver but as an indulgence. Because cash is burning a hole in your pocket, you simply must have that generous slice of New York cheesecake. It goes so well with your cappuccino. Not that you're hungry. You just feel like it. Or because you just got paid for a completed project.

Because you have a redeye flight for work, you find yourself enjoying a sirloin steak close to midnight at one of the airport restaurants. It's a business expense and a way of keeping you awake, so you order away and even get two side dishes for good measure. Project deadline coming up? No worries. Help is on the way in buckets of chicken wings, potato salads, and coleslaw, so clear that conference table pronto. You sit all day at your desk, but no big deal. "Desk work is cerebral work is tiring work. I still burn all those calories somehow." Sure. If you say so.

It's very easy to find excuses to eat. Sugar rush is real. Chips produce a delightful crunch in your mouth. That root beer hits just the right spot at the back of your parched throat. With so much overprocessed foodstuff formulated to keep you coming back for more, you begin to identify it as more than just nourishment. It's a source of pleasure and pleasure is what your innermost being often seeks when you've had a crummy day and need some sort of validation for yourself. With just one tap of a button, it comes conveniently to your doorstep and you can commence to restore some semblance of faith in yourself.

Nowadays, eating food also has a lot to do with visual enjoyment. I'm sure you've heard the expressions "his eyes were bigger than his stomach" or "the see-food diet" and may have even laughed at their use. Funny as they are, the truth behind them are what food companies are counting on to keep you spending on their products. Plating in restaurants is now an artform, as much a part of the gustatory experience as the actual taste itself. It makes you feel good to be surrounded by such aesthetic wonders.

Can't make up your mind on what to eat? Confounded by the million and seven choices on a menu? Have a flight, a little of everything. Without your noticing it, all those tastings add up to some serious calories at the end of dinner. And you can't even burn them at the gym or on your morning park run because you'll simply have no time. Your clique of ladies who brunch are meeting the next day to celebrate somebody's promotion. You're fairly certain that you'll still be too full to eat, but you'll go anyway because you can't say no to your gal pals.

I could go on all day, narrating anecdote after anecdote about how people find reasons to eat beyond survival and sustenance. It's the shape of society today with choices, convenience, cash, and card as part of everybody's way of life. You might even force yourself to eat just because you have another C: a conscience. You clean up your plate because there are people starving somewhere in some remote village thousands of kilometers away from yours.

Now that it's clear that eating has become so much more than just a biological imperative to us humans, the next thing to look into is how our emotions affect it. I had mentioned earlier that food can give you a pleasurable experience when tasted—the sight of it alone can give you very positive feelings. But are these substantive and essential positive feelings? Do they make you become a better human being?

The short answer is no. When you derive "feel-good" feels from food, they're actually negative emotions masquerading as upbeat ones to compensate for something that doesn't sit well inside you—and I'm not talking about the leftovers from two nights ago eaten today. Try opening your cupboards and fridge and see what kinds of food you have. I'm very sure there'll be lots of empty carbs in the pantry: cake mixes, muffins, sugar-coated breakfast cereals, and mac-and-cheese boxes. You and so many others are drawn to sugars and highly refined grains and cereals because the gratification they provide is almost immediate.

According to a university research, the foods you crave (as opposed to those which meet your basic survival needs) are usually connected to whatever emotion has you under its spell at the moment or one you're striving for. When you're ecstatic because your favorite celebrity couple got married, you celebrate with no-brainer pizza delivered right to your doorstep. When you fail to pass the exams for grad school, Ben & Jerry's quickly joins your pity party. When you binge on *The Crown*, bags of barbecue tortilla chips are there to keep your hands preoccupied, while your brain and the rest of your body enter into a state of semiconsciousness. It's almost a predictable matchup of food vis-à-vis activity because salt is for when you're bored; crunch is for when you're frustrated or angry; sweet is for when you're happy; and spice is for when you're excited. The food comes to quiet your emotions. After they fade into the background, you have to contend with the after-math of your craving, which doesn't resemble anything like physical hunger and can simply be a buildup to even crazier cravings.

Physical hunger is easy to deal with. It pokes at you for attention, but you can ignore it. It'll keep trying to catch your attention. Next time, it might try a hard tug at your arm. Or a quick shake of your shoulder. Or a swift kick to your shin. Its entry into your consciousness is gradual, which is why you can postpone it for a bit. It can be satisfied by just about anything you lay on the table. It's not your nit-picky eater. When physical hunger is fed, it stops eating. It doesn't come with a generous helping of guilt to make you feel small.

There's another kind of hunger that's quite predatory and very much unlike physical hunger. Emotional hunger comes at you like a bedraggled stranger that kicks the door in and doesn't wait for a warm welcome. It immediately calls for your attention. It asks you for very specific foodstuff: the mango milk bubble tea by the corner store on Main Street. Even after you provide the desired craving, it still wants more. It can never experience fullness, so you plunge into a pit of deep embarrassment. ("Do you have a bovine-sized stomach?") Emotional hunger buries you in guilt and shame because overindulgence can—sometimes literally— make you want to throw up. Your emotions are a very demanding taskmaster indeed.

Emotional eating is an activity that involves using food as a coping mechanism for your negative feelings. It comes to you in a flash. It can "suddenly dawn on you" that you want to go to a Waffle House at three in the morning. Prior to that, you had spent the whole night tossing and turning, trying to figure out how to pay your student loan. You don't even make the connection that the earlier wrestling match with numbers has something to do with your predawn craving.

Eating your feelings is very specific. You usually want the no-nos: the three-patty burgers, the giant burritos, the three-inch slabs of tricolad. You shove everything into your wide-open mouth and—as you clean off the dessert plate and push back your chair—you're still not quite content. Some friends joke that it's because you have too many worms to feed in your tummy. In truth, it's because emotions are a bottomless pit and need the "right stuff" to fill it. When you're at home alone in your bathroom, looking at yourself in the full-length mirror while standing on the truth-teller aka the weighing scale, you realize that you shouldn't have eaten that much. All these scenarios are what make emotional hunger so different from physical hunger.

While all these sound dire and the stuff of doomsday, the great news for you is that it's never too late to get out of the rut you're in. After you've recognized the problem, the next step is to address the real cause head on. No, it's not your growling tummy. It's your worries and fears running rampant through the corridors of your mind. It's your stress and tension raising your blood pressure and constricting your muscles. Regardless of what shape or size your inner demons are, there is definitely something you can do to vanquish them.

While it's good to know and acknowledge that you're an emotional eater, your work doesn't end there. If you're to avoid the monkey on your back for good, you must also acquaint yourself with what keeps it there as a troublesome presence. As the Chinese philosopher and general, Sun Tzu, intones, "If you know the enemy and know yourself, you need not fear the result of a hundred battles".

Emotional eating doesn't happen in a vacuum. It comes about because something or some things trigger it. Here are a few of them:

- **Stress.** It's the usual suspect cause of a lot of today's medical conditions. It's the spawn of a bullet-train world and a snail-paced human. Stress makes you "hungry" because it produces a hormone called cortisol. Cortisol is needy and demands salt, sugar, and grease as its appearance fee. In return, all those fries and milkshakes transform into pleasure and energy for you. The latter may be short-lived, but the fact doesn't register in your brain. You just want to "feed the beast" and forget about it right now.
- **Emotion suppression.** Nobody likes the "Karens and Kens" of human emotions—the headline-grabbing, loud, disruptive, dramatic emotions like anger, anxiety, fear, sadness, etc. You often resort to eating to keep them quiet

and away from public view, pushed down and hidden somewhere in the folds of your digestive tract. The suppression doesn't last long, of course, but you take what minutes you can because they're better than nothing.

- **Filling the void.** The paradox of today's society is that it's full of materials, products, services, and activities to keep you occupied, but it can still leave you empty and unfulfilled. When that happens, you turn to food to cover up the spaces and "kill time". The ennui and emptiness are not the real culprits but the probable reasons behind their occurrence: feeling unmoored and useless or something along those lines.

- **Childhood patterns.** If you were the child whose parents "bribed" you with ice cream if you went calmly to the dentist for a tooth extraction, then you grow up to become an adult who associates food with "something good". When you're in a post-breakup funk or horribly sad at missing your deceased mom-confidante, you turn to food to capture the good feeling.

- **Social pressure.** You have family, friends, and colleagues who love to gather together for a meal. You never turn an invite down from them because their company makes you extremely happy and forget the car repairs you need to pay for. Because you lose yourself in all that warmth and bonhomie, you lose track of how much you eat and, before you know it, an entire feast for a tiny nation can sit in your stomach for a whole week.

With triggers coming from every direction, it's no surprise that you can barely keep things together for yourself. Emotional eating becomes your default action to their onslaught and you identify yourself as a true-blue emotional eater. It's a tragic confession, but it's a good start toward freedom from it. Anybody familiar with the 12 steps first developed by Alcoholics Anonymous is familiar with this principle. An admission of your problem and helplessness at its power over you is always step one. To deepen your self-knowledge further, here is another list to sift through for the kind of emotional eater that you are:

- Stress eaters try to get rid of the knots in their stomach and shoulder muscles by shoveling food into their mouths like there was no tomorrow. Again, there are plenty of these clips from movies and TV shows. It's comical only when it happens to somebody else. When it's you stress-eating, it's tragic because it's nothing more than a diversion to draw your attention away from your mortgage payment deadline. It does nothing concrete to take care of the looming financial responsibility.

- Unhappy eaters use food as their source of happiness and good cheer. The film cliché of a mascara-stained face gobbling down a tub of ice cream exists because it's founded on reality. An impending divorce is a good excuse. The death of a pet is another. Loneliness needs a pity party and unhappy eaters bring along their friends me, myself, and I to commiserate.
- Rage eaters need food like a shot in the arm to calm them down. It helps them forget how angry they are at the boss who passed them over for a promotion. This possibly explains why there's a huge banquet scene that often follows a massive battle scene in the movies. All that rage has to be channeled toward something that will not entail decapitation or disembowelment.
- Dissatisfied eaters are untethered and adrift on an ocean of the blahs. Nothing seems to be "happening" in their lives, so eating becomes that meaningful activity to keep them busy in their waking hours.

- Festive eaters use every milestone in their lives to celebrate and "celebrate" always equates to scarfing down mountains of food. No viral infection? Drive-thru at McDonald's. First paycheck? Dinner at Olive Garden with the fam. Best friend's engagement? Brunch buffet at a countryside inn. They can't think of any other way to mark special occasions other than to eat —and eat to excess.

Do any of these descriptions (or a combination of them) fit you?

When you let your emotions dictate what, when, where, why, and how you eat, you soon discover that it has serious consequences not just on your weight but on your general health. Experts have established that negative emotions beget negative eating habits. If you're not overeating, you're undereating. There's no in-between for you because that's the nature of emotional eating. You develop a blind side to the middle ground. Like a pendulum, you can swing from one extreme to the other. You then always tend to reach for the "comfort foods".

I mentioned earlier that food companies usually formulate their products in such a way that you get "addicted" to them; this is by deliberate design on their part. They want you to want them. Their food and drinks become comfort food because they're convenient, accessible, cheap, and give you the ingredients you want in excessive quantities: sugar, salt, and the rest of the gang. You especially like licking the crumbs off the foil bag—that's where all the "yummy goodness" is concentrated. The next day, guilt weighs heavily on your mind and you punish yourself by exercising to sheer exhaustion. And because you burned off a whole lot of calories, you have to compensate by eating a lot again—you know, as a reward. This is very traumatic to your pancreas, liver, kidney, heart, etc. Just like any machine, your body undergoes wear and tear, but this abnormal eating behavior is like stepping on the accelerator, speeding up an impending breakdown.

Don't be surprised that you often feel nauseated by the whole bingeing. That's the body's natural reaction to your excesses. Even a tummy ache is to be expected. Payback is always right around the corner because your body can only take so much abuse before it turns on you. If you're not happy with your current body weight, that's very likely not just about genes or DNA—things that may not always be possible to control. But do take a moment to consider that you may actually also be responsible for your unsatisfactory bodily condition. The great thing about that realization? That it's also well within your power to rein it all in. You have the resources to reverse the process. You can correct your own wrongs.

Righting wrongs in this case doesn't mean putting yourself on a diet. Believe it or not, diets often contribute to emotional eating. They appear to be sufficient stop-gap measures, but they're still not addressing the real issues. At best, they provide artificial and temporary solutions by prescribing limits and scopes to your food intake: more protein, less carbs, more "good" fats, less salt, no salt, etc. If only it were that easy. At some point, your mind and body will protest at this indignity. Food is food is food. Don't take it out on inanimate objects. This is similar to the conundrum associated with money. Money itself is neutral, but your love/hate relationship to it is what makes it evil— or useful. Food is not at fault here. It's your relationship to it that makes it friend or foe.

Before we move on to the next chapter, please take time to do the following quiz:

Are You an Emotional Eater?

Check yes if the statement best describes you, your situation, or your reaction. Check no if it doesn't.

1. I eat more than my normal food intake when I'm under stress, e.g., rushing to meet a deadline.❏ Yes ❏ No
2. I browse on whatever food I find on the kitchen counter just because it's there, not because I'm hungry.❏ Yes ❏ No
3. I eat to feel the opposite of whatever I feel at the moment, e.g., sadness to happiness.❏ Yes ❏ No
4. I reward myself with food whenever I reach personal milestones. ❏ Yes ❏ No
5. I eat to the point beyond satiation. ❏ Yes ❏ No
6. Food gives me a sense of security and safety. ❏ Yes ❏ No
7. Food makes me lose all sense of self-control. ❏ Yes ❏ No
8. I can't watch movies at home or at the cineplex without a bucket of popcorn, supersized soda, and hotdogs by my side. ❏ Yes ❏ No
9. I must always eat when I meet friends at a restaurant, even though I may not be hungry at all. ❏ Yes ❏ No
10. I sneak a cookie out of my colleague's drawer when they're not in the office. ❏ Yes ❏ No
11. I make multiple trips to the food table at a friend's birthday party. ❏ Yes ❏ No
12. When I'm bored, I forage through the fridge and pantry for food to eat. ❏ Yes ❏ No

13. I never say no when offered a second helping of my favorite food. ❑ Yes ❑ No
14. I panic when somebody invites me to a special dress-up event because I can't fit into any of my fancy outfits anymore. ❑ Yes ❑ No
15. I resort to bad behavior when I'm under pressure. ❑ Yes ❑ No

If you have answered one, most, or all questions with yes, you may be inclined toward emotional eating. You're off to a good start. Awareness is key. When you know that you hamper your own efforts at weight loss (or gain) because you're a slave to your emotions, you gain a fresh perspective into the issue and can tackle things differently. In this case, you may actually realize that weight loss in itself is not and shouldn't be the end-all, be-all of your journey to health and wellness. There is so much more to aim for than just reducing yourself to a size five. The following chapter provides an alternate view of weight loss.

2

THE PROBLEM WITH
WEIGHT LOSS

Several decades ago, in the late 1970s, a quirky film in the black comedy/murder mystery genre came out called *Who Is Killing the Great Chefs of Europe?* As the title suggests, the best and brightest kitchen masters were being murdered under circumstances similar to how they prepared their signature dishes. After an intense investigation that spanned several countries, the murderer was finally discovered to be the female assistant of a highly respected gourmet magazine publisher. Her love and admiration for her morbidly obese boss—who couldn't say no to food—drove her to take matters into her own hands and kill the very people she blamed for his unfortunate weight.

While the movie isn't quite a weight-loss story, it does drive home the point that weight issues aren't just a recent human obsession (the movie is over four decades old, as of this writing), confined to one particular sex, or a simple problem to be dealt with by slicing, dicing, or mincing away the extra pounds off your body. And they're certainly nobody else's responsibility but yours. You can't hire an assassin to off your villainous fats (or the creators of those villainous fats) just because you're tired of looking at yourself in the mirror.

I've no doubt that you're looking for a permanent solution to your eating and weight problems, which brought you to this book, but I don't have a diet solution to offer you. It's time to consider that diets, regardless of how much science is pinned on them to make them attractive and believable, have a limit to how much transformation they can bring to your body. Hike up your protein intake. Reduce your carbs. Eat like prehistoric hunter-gatherers. They can all drive you insane as you try to keep track of what's good to eat and what's not. There's something seriously out of whack about something that keeps you constantly on edge and guilty about some intangible sin you committed on yourself. Well, it's time to put the troll that makes your life miserable, under a microscope. Let's see if that very noisy monster in your head is worth the time of day you give it. Meet your troll: diet culture.

Diet culture is a belief system that associates being thin with good health and overall well-being. If you're not thin, then something must be wrong with your body, mind, and spirit. It's that worldview that celebrates Barbie, beauty pageants, and skeletal runway models. It makes fun of you for not reaching your size-five target to fit in a bridesmaid's dress for your best friend's wedding. Even though multiple academic and government studies show that diets fail most of the time (either from the get-go or in the post-diet scenario, when you gain back all that you lost and then some), the culture will have you believe that you're simply not trying hard enough.

Diet culture traps you into thinking that you must fit into a particular mold to be acceptable in the world. Like Cinderella's two stepsisters, you struggle to fit into the "glass slipper" of society's measure. It pushes you to be completely dissatisfied with your body's lumps and bumps because you can't jam them into the cinder girl's lost footwear, throwing you into a whirlwind of negative emotions. You're not one of those people who can laugh when someone mocks you about your body shape. "Round is a shape" isn't in your arsenal of repartees. Instead, you take the flight route of the fight-or-flight response.

Despite its bully nature—or maybe because of it—diet culture stands on shaky ground. The fundamental principle of any diet is deprivation. You deprive your body one type of nutrient in favor of another primarily to lose your "excess baggage". Your mind starts parsing the contents of your pantry and fridge to abide by diet guidelines that pronounce one ingredient good; the other, bad.

One time, a friend's elderly mom went overboard with her consumption of beetroot juice—morning, afternoon, evening—because it was supposedly good for women of her age. After several weeks of overindulgence, her pee had turned red and her skin had acquired a purplish stain. However, those weren't even the worst results; she developed kidney stones that had to be surgically removed from her body because of the severe pain they caused. Although this example resides on the extreme end of the spectrum, it does highlight a few things. Despite their "good" intentions, diets can do harm and their first casualty is usually the very target of their do-gooding, your body.

To your body, all six major nutrients (carbohydrates, fat, minerals, protein, vitamins, and water) are essential to its development. The food pyramid can't stand with a block missing. When you get rid of one or the other or more, your body doesn't take kindly to the imbalance. It can alter its functions, processes, and even physiological features just to make up for the deficit. Your body does all this in an effort to save itself, even if it were a lost cause. For example, it's no coincidence that many dieters who skimp on protein end up with low bone density. If you don't give masons cement, gravel, and sand, how do you expect them to build you a sturdy wall that can withstand a hurricane?

When you go on a diet, your body can interpret the change in eating habits as a danger sign and act accordingly. It will slow down your metabolism to preserve your stored nutrients and stretch them to their utmost sustainability and usefulness until things return to normal. This is your body's natural starvation mode kicking in. It doesn't know when it could be fed properly again. It has no idea if the apocalypse had already come, wiping out the global food supply. All it knows is that it can be at risk of dying of hunger, so it hoards what it can from your internal storehouses. Since your body refuses to metabolize your plate of paleo palatable into energy, dieting can achieve the opposite of your target effect: make you look puffy and bloated.

Another way your body fights back is by becoming constipated and/or dehydrated—two immediate and unmistakable symptoms of monkey business going on inside you. It's either you're having too little or too much of something, so you commence soul-searching to figure out which. As the gears and cogs in your brain turn and gain momentum, your mind runs everywhere and soon goes into overdrive—desperate to make things right, desperate to regain control, desperate.

It's not just your physical body that receives the worst brunt of your dieting. It also counts your mind as one of its victims. Because diet culture assaults you with the concept of good food versus bad food, you're forced into a constant position of judgment. Every morsel becomes subject to a moral dilemma. Every grocery purchase must be weighed based on its heavenly virtues or hellish temptations. That's no way to live. Diet culture adds an extra layer of stress and anxiety to your daily life by involving you in a decision-making process you were not meant to make as a human being. You're just supposed to buy ingredients, cook and plate them, and bring them to the table for your meal, not count their grammage on a kitchen scale and scrutinize the fine print of food packages. Every. Single. Time.

As with marriage, dieting has its own honeymoon stage before things start falling apart. You couldn't say no to a colleague's birthday pub crawl. You were too tired to cook, so you ordered and ate a family-size pizza meal from Domino's by yourself. When you find yourself having more cheat days than on-days—because absolutely no person on Planet Earth can claim perfect obedience to rules and regulations—your tendency is to look inward and beat yourself up for your lack of willpower. "I couldn't say no to that cronut behind the glass counter." Once you enter the self-condemnation stage, there's no stopping the avalanche of guilt, shame, depression, and everything in between. It's already exhausting just writing the terms down, how much more living them all.

To cover up your transgression and release some of the tension building up in the pit of your stomach, you adopt dysfunctional behaviors like forcing yourself to throw up, popping diet pills, smoking like a chimney, or gulping down cans of energy drinks. They're all tactics to minimize your food portions or jumpstart your metabolism, but what they're really achieving is to teach your brain to ignore your body. I don't know about you, but that kind of passive-aggressive behavior never flies with me because it's unkind and contemptible. Everybody glares at the mom texting on the phone, while her baby bawls beside her. So why aren't you doing that to yourself when you disregard your body's needs? You're giving it everything else but what it's begging for. In such an unpleasant setting, you drive your body to do the unthinkable: imbibe the worst possible eating disorders—anorexia and bulimia are just two—and focus rabidly on the very foods you're supposed to avoid.

It's impossible to discuss diet culture and dieting without including the subject of weight loss itself. As one of the main reasons for dieting, weight loss has a commanding presence in the minds of dieters. It's meant to be a mantra for pushing away that basket of tacos and racking up thousands of steps on your pedometer. While weight loss may translate to an aesthetically pleasing shape in your view, it may spell the difference in a literal life-or-death medical issue for another. At face value, therefore, weight loss in itself isn't problematic. Where it doesn't stand scrutiny is in the thinking surrounding weight loss.

Weight-loss hopefuls—you may be one of them—often place all their chips on the table, aka the goal, with no room for error, compromise, or other variables. If after three months you still haven't dropped from 150 pounds to 118 pounds to be at your beach body best, then you do away with the whole notion of weight loss altogether. You forget that it has health-related benefits; you're just focused on the fact that some extra pounds are still clinging tenaciously to your body.

You may not see it when you stand in front of the mirror, but you've already shed a noticeable amount of weight. Even your mother-in-law compliments you for it and your hairstylist admires your now-visible cheekbones. However, you register none of it because you're obsessed about your unachieved target weight. You abandon all the positive strides you've made, and your 130-pound self cries out, "I'm done with losing weight. I'm simply incapable of getting down to 118."

You view your deficit of 12 pounds as a failure, while the rest of the world celebrates the 20 pounds you lost. It's such a twisted perspective, but that's a common train of thought among weight-loss wannabes. The despair then develops into an overlying concept that your good health and coveted weight are not meant for you. You don't deserve to be hale and happy. You should learn to live with how you are now and don't bother other people about it. Move on. *C'est la vie.*

When you dissect the insides of that despair, you realize that it can stem partly from your desire to have quick fixes. You want a fairy godmother who can just wave her wand and transform you into a lithe figure in the blink of an eye. It can also emanate from your unconscious belief that losing weight can solve a host of other problems. "My partner won't leave me if I lose weight." "I'll be a more productive member of society if I lose the weight I put on over Christmas," forgetting that you've been unemployed for weeks now and unwilling to hit the pavement in search of a job.

"Losing weight will help me live with myself." You put so much significance and credence into weight loss that it's a miracle it hasn't gone on its own weight-loss program for all the baggage you have piled on it.

If weight loss becomes the driving force of your every waking hour because you want to stop people from talking smack about you, then you need to pump the brakes, slow down, and re-evaluate your situation. The worst thing you can do to yourself is to use other people's negative views about you to fuel your weight loss. In such a scenario, you put them in the driver's seat, leaving you with no control over your life. You might just end up compounding your physical problem with mental ones because dwelling on other people's negativity can create such a deep darkness in your mind and soul.

You may also be one of those people, who asserts control over your circumstances by expecting nothing less than perfection in everything that you do. You believe that somewhere out there is a firmly established ideal shape and size for your body, and you're destined to pursue your very own golden aesthetic. You pronounce that ideal as the key to utopia, which—when achieved—guarantees you eternal joy, the love that you deserve, and the bliss that is worth the whole world to you.

With your weight-loss program propelled by your drive for perfection, you leave no room for your own human frailties. You may not like the sound of "your own human frailties", but it's the truth. We all have it. If you still haven't shed the targeted 25 pounds by Thanksgiving, you must be able to say it's okay, shrug it off, and resolve to do better. Or move on and aim for something else. But the thing is, if you're a perfectionist, it's mortal sin to fall short of your goal. When that happens, you may not know how to cope.

At this point, it's important to love yourself enough to let go of such a notion as perfection. (Cue Queen Elsa's anthem.) It's not gonna happen at any time in your entire life, not because you're fundamentally inutile but because you're human. To fail—sometimes spectacularly—is part of your job description. When you can calibrate your mindset to accept that, you can make better and more realistic plans that won't stress you out or make you feel like a perennial failure.

The thing about perfection is that it can actually be a deterrent to your weight-loss plans. You may be one of those perfectionists, who freezes in one spot (yes, still an Elsa pun) when you suddenly realize that success is not guaranteed. Because you've been advised by a medical doctor that losing 10 pounds in one month at your age is risky, you forget about the whole weight-loss thing altogether. You didn't notice that you could have actually adjusted your plans so that instead of 10 pounds you could just target four pounds to lose in a month. Perfectionism breeds the mindset of "my way or the highway", so you're not going to adjust your expectations or goals any time soon. Meanwhile, you lose an opportunity to get rid of four pounds.

This leads to another issue when embarking on a weight-loss journey: self-sabotage, where you are your own worst enemy. You may be dropping pounds and inches regularly over the course of a few weeks. You're feeling very good about yourself for your consistency. To give yourself a reward, you declare "a rare cheat day" to indulge in a half-dozen donuts—you can't help yourself; you're happy. Before you know it, you also find a reason to skip your daily stretching exercise and other activities related to losing weight. When it suddenly hits you that you've been very remiss in keeping your commitment, guilt starts to consume you and you label yourself a loser. At that point, you simply embrace your inability to lose weight as a fact of life and move on, never to get up and try again.

Self-sabotage arises from one or more factors. Besides your inability to manage your emotions (and eat them), it may stem from a lack of self-confidence or self-worth. You may be doing great in the first few days or weeks of your regimen, but the progress is very slow. You question your power to do the long haul because it may entail giving up so much. "And why the heck am I punishing myself?" You start viewing your regimented eating as undeserved punishment for "inherited genes that make me gain weight in the first place". So, the house of cards that is your weight-loss program comes crashing down. It's almost like you're afraid of success. You stop just short of your goal because you don't know what to do with yourself once you attain your target weight. On the other hand, your fear of failure prompts you not even to try it.

Weight loss is a great goal and your desire to do it is something worth following through. I'm the first one to cheer you on to undertake it. As you prepare yourself physically to get into a weight-loss plan, don't forget to prepare yourself mentally as well. You want and need to approach weight loss with the right mindset. You should strive to be the person who sets realistic expectations of yourself. You avail yourself of the best information to help you with your goal-setting. Above all, you want to be your own best friend.

Being your own best friend within the context of a weight-loss program means you learn to accept your shortcomings and weaknesses. Perfectionism has no place in an activity that may have as many downs as ups, like a rollercoaster ride. You shouldn't keep doubting yourself and negating the progress you've already accomplished. Don't be your worst enemy; love yourself and let yourself fail sometimes. It's what living is all about.

Beyond the pep talk, what I really want to say to you is this: Dieting is not the answer to your current issues with eating and weight loss. For the real root of the problem, you need to look deeply into how you manage your emotions and allow your thoughts to flow. Emotions and thoughts may be intangible things, but they affect a lot of the outward aspects of your life. If you can learn to deal with them in suitable ways so that steer you clear of unhealthy habits and choices that they create, you may just find yourself on track to succeed without the stress and harassment from your inner demons, aka the perfectionist, the self-saboteur, and the self-hater.

In succeeding chapters, you'll have the opportunity to know more about the LET GO Method that may unlock the doors for transforming your mind (metaphorically responsible for your thoughts) and heart (same but for your emotions). It's an acronym that stands for the following key concepts:

- Lead Your Thoughts
- Evade Your Triggers
- Tune in to Your Emotions
- Give in to Your Real Needs
- Observe and Obey Your True Hunger

The main goal in acquainting yourself with them is to give you leadership over your life. I'm not using the word "control" here because you don't want to picture yourself as some sort of extreme dictator, without any compassion and kindness for yourself. You want to influence your emotions and thoughts in such a way that it builds up your self-confidence and helps you to love yourself better, not pressure you to the point of breaking or burnout or worse. With that in mind, let's move on to the first concept: Lead Your Thoughts.

3

LEAD YOUR THOUGHTS

In the childhood fairy tale of Snow White and the seven dwarfs, if the evil stepmother desired a dose of truth-telling, she always turned to her magic mirror, which did not hold back from its pronouncements—sometimes at risk to its own life and limb, so to speak. Since no such supernatural fixture has made itself known in the real world just yet, you're left to trust other people and yourself to dish out the truth, when you need to hear it. The only problem with this arrangement is that—as the main character of House, M.D., regularly declares—everybody lies, including you to yourself.

One of the biggest lies you can say to yourself involves your physical appearance. "My self-confidence and self-worth are intrinsically woven into how I look." There is a direct correlation to the billion-dollar fashion, fitness, and wellness industries and your personal need to look stunning. In many cases, your interpretation of stunning translates to a svelte figure that pours effortlessly into the sample sizes (zero to two) of the fashion houses of the world—despite the fact that, in recent years, more plus-size people strut their stuff on the red carpet and own it.

To become a lithesome form, you sweat, stretch, spin, starve, and supplement yourself to kingdom come. No superfood is safe from your radar because you must achieve that gap between your thighs or else. In the meantime, society keeps piling on the lies about your face, chest, belly, and bottom. After a while, they're all that you hear, making you anxious about your looks and obsessive about how others view you. In your own eyes, your body becomes nothing but an object to evaluate for its parts being in their proper places and in proportion to the rest of you.

What the world may have to say about your body— whether it's a compliment about how firm your arms look in that tank top or a diss from your weighing scale after adding five pounds in as many days—doesn't matter. They're just words. It's not your life purpose to adjust accordingly to their standards. Your mantra for weight loss shouldn't be "Once I'm x pounds, the bouncer at the club will not look at me with judge-y eyes." "When I hit my goal weight, I'll literally feel lighter and figuratively walk on cloud nine." "If I maintain my current size, my partner won't ever leave me for somebody else." That's giving way too much power to people other than yourself. Someone else is piloting your journey and it's not you.

Weight can never and should never be the measure of your worth. That's a sure-fire way of ensuring your unhappiness. As with a lot of human characteristics, it's not stable enough to be reliable. Trust Thanksgiving and Christmas Day to nudge the needle of the weighing scale upward. Weight is also quite relative, even depending on some of the most fundamental laws of physics. If you really want to appear feathery, you may want to sign up for the space program to explore Mars. With the Red Planet's lesser gravity pull, you'll be a wisp in the war god's domain.

What doesn't change is your mass. It's not affected by gravity, speed, and all the clothes, makeup, and hair products you wear. The same is true with your self-worth. A drill sergeant can dress you down, a nephew can poke at the folds of your belly and laugh, a colleague can tease you for the front buttons of your business shirt popping out, but none of them and their words can and should touch the value of your personhood. External factors have nothing to do with your self-worth; its price tag is established inside you by you.

A low self-worth means you view yourself as undeserving of any kind of investment in time and effort. It's too much to ask of yourself to try to lose weight. What for? You see nothing, anything beyond yourself, which could make your life worth something, worth the investment in athleisure wear. You don't feel compelled to push yourself beyond your limit because you don't see the point. It won't change the negative view people have of you. No one has your back, so why take the risk of injuring yourself or getting sick as you try to better your physical body?

When you nurture a low self-worth, it can spell trouble for your weight and whatever plans you have for losing some of it or gaining more. If you do attempt, say, a weight-loss program, you don't set SMART (specific, measurable, achievable, realistic, and time-bound) goals. Maybe out of frustration because of the constant harassment of your siblings, you sort of wave your hand in the air and say, "Yeah, yeah. Fine. I'll lose weight." And that's the extent of your commitment to it. Your heart is not in it, so you're not motivated to set it up so there can be follow-through, accountability, and ownership.

Even after you make that vague commitment to do something about your weight, nothing concrete comes out of it. You said it just to get people off your back, not actually to do it. Since you don't value yourself and believe others don't either, the notion of trying to be healthier or better seems an utter waste of resources. You feel more satisfaction indulging all night on chips and dips, compounding your weight issues further.

If by some miracle, a near-and-dear steps in to intervene and ensure your compliance to a weight goal, you still go about doing it with no vested interest. Everything you put into it will be mediocre. You won't end up developing good habits from the exercise, just an abiding frustration at the bulldog near-and-dear, watching your every move. The moment the smallest failure or delay or mistake happens, you abandon ship and classify the whole experience as "never to be repeated again".

"Wow! Your partner must really love you to devote so much effort into looking good." A mark of low self-worth is when you do what you do for others and not for yourself. Everybody else deserves the best of you except you, so you launch into a spasm of dieting and exercising to keep other people happy. When you finally reach your goal, the result seldom lasts long. If the people to whom you dedicated your weight loss change in their demeanor toward you and discard you like last week's leftovers, your old weight is almost guaranteed to come back, bringing with it new friends.

Your low self-worth can also keep you too busy to take care of yourself. You willingly work overtime and use it as an excuse to skip a meal or your exercise time. You prioritize a friend's need over your own need, so you juggle your schedule to accommodate them, setting aside the time meant for your weight-loss regimen.

Everybody else is doing well in their weight-loss program except you—or so you figure out from constantly monitoring the progress of other people. Your own doesn't feel as important. You focus on others and compare theirs to your negligible advancement. They seem to be doing so much better than you. You don't even have a cheerleader to pep you up because the relationships you've surrounded yourself with are all toxic. Your low self-worth allowed you to settle ... for the verbally abusive, the cruel jokers, the exploiters, etc.

In the end, you won't even make yourself accountable to anyone else. You know you're floundering, but you don't cry out for help. You don't create for yourself an atmosphere conducive to success by lining up caring people to become part of a support group of sorts. Instead, you draw farther away from others and inward into yourself. It scares you that they'll say and do hurtful things to you once you make yourself vulnerable to them. They might just complicate your insecurities further, so never mind. Your low self-worth continues and you have no one around to speak the truth to you about how you matter. Meanwhile, you develop a harsher view of yourself and conditions like body dysmorphia make you your worst critic. You notice your every bodily flaw. You stare at the mirror and see a beached walrus, pushing you in the direction of eating disorders.

The longer you stay in the neighborhood of low self-worth, the easier it is for you to learn the worst possible habits, one of which is negative self-talk. If you've ever watched the classic TV series, *The Muppet Show*, then you know Statler and Waldorf, the two loud and tetchy elderly hecklers up on the theatre balcony. From their high and mighty vantage point, they are always quick to voice their displeasure and criticism at every bungle and blooper made by the actors on stage. For the general viewership, of course, they kind of tone down the wording they use to make fun of other muppets. You, however, in the privacy of your thoughts, do not hold back from using the harshest words to kill all that is good inside you.

Negative self-talk shrouds you in an atmosphere of gloom and doom. Every "idiot, loser, failure, etc." you pronounce upon yourself reverberates over and over again until all that you hear in your head are those words. The worst result of those deafening, negative words? You begin to believe the lies. You see yourself as incapable of positive development. The most trivial mistakes you make in your weight-loss journey are magnified into mortal sins. "This is why I shouldn't have started this stupid eating schedule. I could never remember which is what for this day and time! I'm such a loser." "If I can't even say no to an acquaintance's invite to all-you-can-eat Thursdays, how do I expect to stick to the weight-loss plan for my best friend's wedding? I'm done with this nonsense. I'd rather die full than hungry. I'm such an idiot to think I can change myself."

Negative self-talk is the opposite of cheerleading and pep talks. It steals your willpower, drains your energy, and blinds you to your true self-worth. It tells you no every time you attempt to change for the better. As negativity takes over your thoughts, you become prone to overeating or starvation—pick your poison— according to how you feel. Yes, that's eating your emotions in action once again. Close at the heels of or side by side with emotional eating could be depression or anxiety. How could you not feel either or both when you seem unable to succeed at anything? What's the point of living, right?

Without any reason to keep on thriving, the dominos of your life start falling one after the other. Anything related to your weight-loss journey—grocery shopping at a health-food store instead of Costco and its super-sized food packages, an hour's exercise three times a week at the nearby gym, a full eight-hour sleep—all become casualties, buried and forgotten in the grave-yard of your nonstarters and best intentions. You feel nothing even in their absence because nothing moti-vates you anymore. You've given up on yourself and life.

Although you've now entered terrifyingly dire straits, there's always a chance to reverse things and the power to do that lies in your hands. You fell into the worst possible habits because you kept following the same patterns of thinking and acting over a significant period until they became as natural to you as breathing. With cognitive restructuring, you dismantle the bad parts of the said patterns and rebuild them into better ones or create new ones altogether.

Cognitive restructuring isn't some new-fangled psychobabble; it's the core of cognitive behavioral therapy (CBT), which has been around since the 1960s. It has remained valid and useful to this day because it works. A therapist and a patient come together to help the latter identify ways of thinking within themselves that contribute to and compound their current woes. Once the patient has recognized them, the therapist and patient work together to reorganize those problematic thought patterns and transform them into something productive and beneficial to the patient. Within the context of this book, you learn to look honestly and deeply into yourself to understand what births perfectionism, low self-worth, negative self-talk, and other inner demons. Your main goal is to steer your thoughts and emotions in a direction that allows you to develop in a positive way. In short, it's all about undoing your self-troll tendencies and getting with the program to eat better, lose (or gain) weight, and become a healthier, better human being.

One way of accomplishing the transformation is by self-monitoring. Notice the details surrounding the occasions when you troll yourself about your eating habits or weight. I have a cousin who goes into panic mode every time a wedding comes up. "I won't be able to fit into anything! And then I end up going to the wedding in my dowdiest dress and sitting in a corner with zero invites to dance." From that point, everything goes downhill because she then starts hating the fact that she can't say no to any type of cake or pastry. She bewails the fact that she never has time to hit the gym because she has to pick up extra shifts at the diner to take care of her son and herself. Sometimes, it's not a wedding but a baby shower or a class reunion, or Thanksgiving dinner. Any time there's a big gathering, when people are expected to gussy up a bit, mix and mingle in a sea of friends and strangers alike, and eat and make merry, my cousin melts down. Her biggest anxiety is that people will treat her like she doesn't belong there. She feels her height (five feet, 11 inches) and weight (over 200 pounds), so she can't even make herself invisible or small. She thinks that dressing up for such events is an exercise in futility. Regardless of what she wears, she's just a blimp in drapery, according to her.

It's useful to monitor these occurrences, so you can prepare yourself. If need be, have pen and paper, or a device ready to record every time you castigate yourself over your body. Awareness creates an opportunity for you to change. The journal you write doesn't have to contain Pulitzer-level essays. Every notation can be something as simple as bullet points on what you felt and thought at the moment you trolled yourself. If you don't know what triggered your negative self-talk, write down that fact. If you know the trigger, expound on it. If your surroundings have a bearing on your negativity, jot down details.

The more you monitor and write down your moments of unkindness to yourself, the easier it is for you to discover the set patterns. Once you bring them to the light, there's no hiding them anymore. Give them a long hard look and establish ways that you can avoid them. If they may seem inevitable, find ways that you can alter them to become positive patterns.

As soon as my cousin realized that preparing for gatherings triggered all her feelings of insecurity about her weight and height, she made sure that she never prepped by herself and her lonesome. It was in her loneliness that she especially felt bitter about herself. Instead, she began to dress up for an occasion always with one of her cheerleaders, aka a cousin aka me, someone who had nothing but positive things to say about her and the way she carried herself. The change was gradual, but she slowly came out of the funk she was in and embraced her size XL shape. Eventually, she did start losing weight but for the right reasons that were meaningful and uplifting to her.

Another technique for turning your negativity into positivity is to question your beliefs, especially about yourself. Not everything you say to yourself is correct, but you won't know it unless you ask yourself the right questions. If you believe yourself to be a fat loser every time you consume a tub of ice cream in one sitting, then evaluate what just happened:

- Is my thinking that I'm a fat loser based on truth or just something triggered because I feel bad about something else, which led to my ice cream bingeing?
- How do I test the correctness of my answer to the first question?
- What should my reaction be if my belief (I'm a fat loser) turns out to be true? What if it's false? What if there's a gradation of grey between those two possible answers?

There's no limit to the questions you can ask yourself. The act of questioning breaks the rhythm of the blows you land on yourself, much like what happens when you shout at a bully to distract them from lunging at somebody's lunchbox. By asking yourself questions, you learn to be more mindful (thoughtful) about yourself. You might even learn to be kind to and love yourself as you uncover hidden gems about your life. Your questions help you diagnose some of the difficulties you're facing. You realize that your ice cream bingeing wasn't the root of the problem; it was just your coping mechanism. The real issue was that you didn't know how to deal with the loss of your job. From that point, continue asking yourself more questions. Don't be surprised that, in your line of questioning, you may come upon a viable solution to address your emotional eating—or anything else that causes you to hate your body and the way you eat.

Evidence gathering is another technique for changing your mental and emotional patterns. In the same journal you created for self-monitoring, jot down details about people, places, things that reinforce or counter beliefs about yourself. If, for instance, you don't want to begin a weight-loss regimen because you just know that you're going to fail at it anyway, write down memories of when you did succeed at something, anything. It doesn't have to be a Nobel Prize. It can be as simple as finishing a CPR course or planning the 25th-anniversary celebration of your parents. You had started something and seen it to its completion. You can achieve the same for losing weight. You just have to begin.

Conducting a cost-benefit analysis of your behavior is another way of transforming your negativity into something positive. If you keep calling yourself a gluttonous blimp, what does it accomplish? Does it produce a good or bad outcome? Does the derogatory phrase have a long-term effect on you? Does it make you a better human being? It's good to keep a firm hand on the words you pronounce on yourself because they can have the power to make or break you. If you feed yourself lies that you're a quitter, you're bound to lose all hope of ever reaching your target weight. But if you bombard yourself with reminders of projects and tasks you've completed, your brain inclines toward the good and you can stop wallowing in the smack talk you've been giving yourself.

One last technique to consider for cognitive restructuring is the generation of alternatives. Look at yourself and your situation with a fresh pair of eyes. If you give in to a family-size bag of potato chips while watching Netflix, don't start beating yourself up with the label "no-good lazy slob of a pig". That harshness should never have any place in your life. Instead, thoughtfully consider the circumstances that led to it. Maybe you could have poured just a small portion of chips into a bowl and kept the rest of the bag in the pantry. That's a lesson learned and something to apply in the future. One night of losing control over food doesn't condemn you for eternity as a greedy glutton. Every day that the sun rises again is another opportunity to do better. Never treat your mistakes as the end of the world. Be thoughtful and kind to yourself.

This leads to another important method of countering all the negativity in your life, especially pertaining to food, eating, and your body image. Practice self-validation. Bad times happen to all of us, but what separates us from each other is how we react to them. A significant part of your reaction can be managed by valuing yourself. You can start by writing down all the people, places, things, and activities that matter to you and explaining why. I'm going to bet that food may not even occupy any of the top spots. You might focus on your parents, siblings, your fluffy rescue, a kids' charity, rollerblading, walking through the woods, etc. When the bad comes bulldozing its way into your life, fall back into all that matters to you. Don't mope alone in the darkness of your room, just 10 feet away from your full pantry and refrigerator. Go out with your dog and enjoy the sunshine and cool breeze around a lake. Invite a friend to play ping-pong with you at the local Y.

An alternative to spending time with the things that matter to you is devoting it to things that you're really good at. Garden. Paint. Sing. Detail your own or a family member's car. Play the drums. All that is far better than indulging in food and feeling the weight of guilt in your entire body afterward. In a sense, you're affirming that you are more than the food you eat. You are more than the shape of your body. When you validate other aspects of your life as a human being, you can live a positive, more holistic life.

When you hear me repeat "be kind to and thoughtful toward yourself", what I'm really encouraging you to do is to practice self-compassion. It's all about forgiving yourself when you fall short of your daily targets for exercise and mindful eating. It's focusing on your journey—the pound a week lost and never returned—rather than the target weight that still seems so far away. It's refraining from throwing every cuss word at yourself for falling into temptation with a large pan pizza all to yourself. It's about formulating lessons learned after slacking off from exercising for a month. The examples for self-compassion are endless. And so should be the patience and understanding that you show yourself. "You're only human" shouldn't be an excuse but a reminder that erring is part of your existence.

In exercising self-compassion, one important technique to learn is H. A. L. T., which stands for Hungry, Angry/Anxious, Lonely, Tired. Let's say you've just come home from work after midnight. Upon passing by the kitchen for a glass of water, you discover a pan of gooey lasagne on the counter, with a note from your partner, which says, "Help yourself." You've already had dinner in the corporate boardroom, courtesy of the bigwigs who needed you to work overtime for a project. The pasta dish looks so scrumptious and it's been a few hours since that fast-food dinner. What do you do? The best approach is to stand back for a few moments before deciding by using H. A. L. T. as a framework. What do you feel that very moment? Even if you're actually hungry, consider the time that it strikes you. It's already almost one in the morning. A third of a banana might be better than a whole plate of lasagne. If you're feeling any of the other three, then it's not food that you need. Go to bed instead and have a full breakfast when you wake up. Food isn't always the solution to what you're feeling at any given moment.

Emotional eating, a poor body image, and all the hurtful thoughts you say to yourself about both shouldn't dominate your mind. You are still in the driver's seat. Lead your thoughts toward a healthy regard for food and your body, and you can approach your health and well-being plans with a better mindset. Henry Ford, founder of the Ford Motor Company, once said, "Whether you think you can or you think you can't, you're right." That's how commanding your thoughts are in your life.

A concrete way of transforming your negative mental and emotional patterns into positive ones is to expose yourself each day to affirmations. Affirmations are words strung together to create a short, positive statement that could influence your thinking for the better. As I mentioned earlier, words have power and affirmations are words that harness that power especially to bring constructive, encouraging, and life-sustaining truths into your existence.

To close out this chapter, I'm sharing some affirmations below for you to read. Set aside time each day to marinate on them and see how best they can make a positive impact in your day-to-day living. To make that happen, it's important that you're confident in their efficacy and the results they bring. Your day's activities and how you conduct them should uphold each affirmation. And do try reading affirmations regularly.

Affirmations

1. I love and respect myself.
2. I'm a work in progress, a masterpiece in the making.
3. I'll never give up.
4. I believe in myself and my ability to succeed.
5. Everything I eat nourishes and strengthens my body and mind.
6. I can and will not be afraid to say no, when needed.
7. I love to exercise and enjoy the body that results from exercising.
8. I have the power to achieve my target weight.
9. I get enough exercise, nourishment, and rest.

10. I'm becoming a better human being every day.

11. I'm winning by exercising every day.

12. My body is beautiful and love everything about it.

13. I enjoy fruits and vegetables as nourishment for my body.

14. Being physically active makes my body feel better.

15. I eat healthy food to feel fit and energetic.

16. Food is not my enemy but an essential, healing, and nurturing element in my life.

17. I'm worthy of all the love in the world.

18. I'm a complete human being in every way.

19. I eat for nourishment and strength each day.

20. Life begins today and every day, not when you reach your target weight.

4

EVADE YOUR TRIGGERS

I f you can step out of your body for a few minutes and observe the times when you eat your feelings or initiate cheat days or binge on all the Pringles flavors in one sitting, it's very likely that you'll notice a pattern emerging. Humans are creatures of habit; you are unlikely to be exempt unless your DNA does classify you as something other than a Homo sapiens. There are no nasty surprises when you let food take the driver's seat in your life. That's the reason why there are such things as triggers—people, objects, situations, emotions, thoughts, etc. that cause you to give in to food and let it control you. They're well-defined as far as you're concerned. They're specific to you; others might have their own set. You give in to your triggers—often quite easily, without putting up a fight. Your triggers could be either internal (something coming from inside you) or external (something coming from outside you).

One of the most common triggers is **social** in nature. You've just left home after a lovely breakfast of overnight oats and a home-brewed cappuccino to meet your friends at a corner café. You pre-empt any invites by telling them that you've just had breakfast, as you join them at their table. It's almost as if they don't hear you because they soon start shoving portions of their orders onto an extra plate, brought in by a waiter for you. You feel guilty about wasting food and offending your friends that you end up gobbling down what is essentially a second breakfast—as though you were a hobbit on a mission to reach Mordor.

Social pressure is real. It comes from other people— some even well-meaning ones like your grandma who thinks you're too scrawny. She can make you feel like a schmuck if you try to refuse a thick strip of bacon, so you eat what she puts in front of you. While you smile gamely through the chews and gulps, your inside is in turmoil—and I'm not just talking about your tummy. You feel trapped and maybe even resentful, but you don't know how to call out for help or how to make them stop.

Another trigger can be **emotional**. Left to their own devices, your emotions can run rampant in the playground of your mind and mess you up. Some of the more roguish emotions are anger, anxiety, ennui, fear, happiness, loneliness, sadness, and timidity. They're always inclined toward making you choose and do the wrong thing. Take anger, for instance. When you're angry, you have bile building up inside you because an unreasonable boss wants you to work overtime to finish a project. That bile is actually a lot of pent-up chaotic energy that's seeking a way out, a way to vent. You're a volcano about to erupt and you channel all that negative force into scarfing down a pound of cheeseburger and knocking it all back with a super-sized tumbler of Coke. You think it's a better alternative to screaming at the jefe to shove the project up where the sun don't shine.

With such a hard slave master … er … taskmaster like this boss, it's no surprise that you can develop loads of anxiety and stress. They can lead you in the direction of the fridge or pantry because they cause your body to secrete an appetite-increasing hormone. Cortisol creates in you a craving for ingredients that especially make junk food hard to resist with their many grams of fat, salt, or sugar. "Have a break, have a KitKat" isn't just a catchy slogan. It can be an invitation to step away from stressors and eat a snack that produces serotonin, a neurotransmitter that gives you happy feels. This is why anxiety is such a powerful trigger to get you eating.

Ennui or boredom forms something like an idle mind, which your elders probably warned you about as the devil's workshop. You cast about for something—anything—to do on a rainy night when the lights are out and even your phone is dead. After crisscrossing your abode, all you can find is a tray of fudge brownies. And so, you indulge yourself. You don't have the energy or desire to think beyond eating food as a time filler. It's an easy choice because the supply is readily available, accessible, and usually doesn't require further action to it, unless you feel the urge to do a Dominique Crenn and earn your own four Michelin stars.

Food seems to be an effective distraction to some people who are prone to fear. You chomp quickly through a bucket of popcorn while watching a horror film because the action keeps you from jumping out of your skin. Eating prevents you from becoming overly invested in the next Pennywise victim's tragic mistake by drawing your attention to the creamy taste of melted cheese instead. Food deflects the blood and gore away from your immediate periphery. It silences the horror by keeping your mind preoccupied with many other things besides the scenes unfolding onscreen.

Emotional eating doesn't just happen in the doom and gloom. You eat a ton of food when you're happy, too. You call it a well-earned celebration, but your physiology calls it doubling the euphoria with the release of dopamine, a happy hormone. Either way, your happiness can be just as much a trigger as the earlier (rather soul-dampening) emotions.

Feelings of loneliness, sadness, and timidity (that is, the lack of self-esteem) also activate your internal feeding frenzy because they require tastes, smells, sights, and textures that fill gaps, raise spirits, and nurture your sense of well-being. I've described a few scenarios in earlier pages when these feelings overwhelm you. You can't really avoid them because they happen to everyone from time to time. The key is learning how to deal with them without them ruining good eating habits.

Besides social pressure and emotions, you may also have **situational or environmental** triggers. You have three square meals a day plus two or three snack breaks not because you're actually hungry but because this pattern has been deeply ingrained in you since childhood. As soon as it's noon, you must have lunch. When four o'clock strikes, you should have tea and cake. I could almost set my watch according to your routines. You don't even think about it anymore. You glide into the office or home pantry at the set time, on autopilot.

Sometimes, a simple close proximity to a food source might lure you in. You walk past a pastry shop exuding the aroma of fresh-baked croissants and you're inside its premises in three seconds flat. Are you hungry? No, but it doesn't matter. That smell is too hard to resist and you will always have space in your tummy for a Danish.

It's also challenging to say no to your food binge when your **mental** and **physiological** states are unstable. Every time your mind goes into dark alleys, thinking about yourself and your lack of worth, it's a short waddle to the kitchen to find something that can cover up all that negativity. If you're constantly worrying about bills and your kids' health or are pregnant and "eating for two", then you can find yourself imbibing an unwanted and unpleasant eating behavior. It's not just the "pregnant phase" of a woman's physiology that can cause her to have crazy cravings; there are premenstrual syndrome and menopause, too. Some conditions like diabetes, Graves disease, and hyperthyroidism can also affect the appetites of not just women but men as well.

If all that you do is wallow in the misery brought about by your triggers, then they can definitely appear daunting, scary, and too numerous to count. However, just because they can ambush you from various directions doesn't mean you should surrender to them in defeat every time. You can still change the whole situation and gain mastery over them. Stripping them of their influence over you begins by **identifying your specific triggers**. It's never one-size-fits-all for them. They are nuanced to fit each individual. Your own trigger or set of triggers is unique to your personality.

The best method of identifying your triggers is to pay attention to the situations that drive you in the direction of the nearest food stash. Note—literally write down—what sort of situations these are. When they happen, you need to be more conscious of your thoughts and emotions and how they flow, of your body and how it behaves. Is it *The Howard Stern Show* in your mind? What is the theme of all the jabbering in your head? How does the mental podcast make you feel? Does your body break out in rashes, cold sweat, stomach cramps, or some other manifestation of disease?

Let's say you've just finished a work project after pulling off some impossible moves behind the scenes to get it all done. You're over the moon about the outcome and can't wait for your boss to say something about it during your team meeting. Instead of giving you even just a small pat on the back, she overlooks the import of the achievement and merely checks it as another item off her list. It's just business as usual for her.

Meanwhile, you're fuming inside because you spent many nights on overtime and missed a few family gatherings, seemingly all for nothing. Not that you expect your boss to fawn over you. A simple kudos would have done the trick. All you can think of at that moment is a side trip to the supermarket for three extra-large pizzas with all the trimmings and a whole gallon of chocolate ice cream to counter the savory goodness of the main meal. You may share it with your family at home, but your mind is convinced that it's mostly for you. You're throwing a party for yourself if no one else is doing it. You know gorging yourself on that much food is a bad idea, but you're going full steam ahead with it because no one else celebrates your invaluable contribution to the world.

Once you recognize a circumstance that makes you want to be a glutton for carbs and realize that the thoughts, feelings, and actions that result from it don't make you love yourself more, you need to follow the trail back to the real root of your behavior, as you would any other mystery. Is it really about your thankless job and stoic boss that you want to eat yourself to oblivion? Or is it something that goes beyond them, perhaps to an earlier time in your life, when you faced a similar situation, an indifference to your best efforts?

Sometimes, a historical review of your life doesn't immediately give you a clear perspective. You may be too close to the situation, giving you a wide blind side. Too many things may be hidden or blurry because you've never processed your past. When that happens, you need to step back and find a better way to view it. An effective approach to understanding the whole scenario—triggers, thoughts, emotions, etc.—is curiosity. You shouldn't pretend that it never happened; you shouldn't try to sweep it aside and hope that it becomes a forgotten moment. It's also not good to face it head-on in a *Clash of the Titans* scene. "Releasing the Kraken" only serves to escalate the situation. You don't come out swinging to fight the circumstance and everything within it—yourself and other people most of all. Rather than taking either of the extreme attitudes, you should shine a light on the situation and try to discern the details surrounding your emotions. Find the similarities, the repeated particulars. Look out for patterns. Behind these repetitions could be the origin story of your emotional eating.

It may very well be that your boss's lack of positive feedback to your accomplishment isn't really what bothers you. It hurts you because it echoes your own parents' lack of validation of your childhood and adolescent milestones. Instead of cheering your salutatorian finish in high school, they grumbled that you didn't make it as valedictorian. Everything you did always seemed to fall short of their measure. And you never stopped trying to get them to notice, even way into your adulthood. It may be a sad discovery for you, but it's a solid beginning toward the next step in the process of overcoming.

Your trigger identification exercise can especially be effective if you keep a journal of everything related to your eating issues. You can call it a food diary, an eating journal—anything, really—for as long as you use it. I mentioned about journaling in earlier chapters of this book and I want to expound further about its efficacy. It's a great tool for dealing with stressful situations; your struggle with food and eating is certainly one. By describing the situation in detail and expounding on your thoughts and emotions at that very moment, in writing, you distance yourself from it. You allow yourself a chance to reflect upon the scenario, evaluate your subsequent actions and reactions, and consider future decisions to make.

One very important aspect about journaling is its ability to show you patterns. As you write down the same types of details over and over again each time they occur, the repetitions emerge; the relationships between circumstances and your responses to them start taking on a tangible shape. Writing down essential details connected to your eating habits and everything about it is a lot like adjusting the magnification of microscope lenses all the minutiae come into sharp focus. The revelation can be startling—maybe even shocking—but a welcome development on the road to overcoming emotional eating.

Besides writing down a general description of how a situation leads you to binge on the contents of your fridge, here are important details to note in your journal:

- The food you ate or wanted to eat
- The who, what, when, where, why, and how of the circumstance that led you to binge on food or made you want to binge on food
- Your thoughts and feelings just before you ate or just before you contemplated bingeing
- Your thoughts and feelings during your bingeing or as you considered food in response to the circumstance
- Your thoughts and feelings after you ate or after you put your contemplation on food behind you

The information you provide can be written as simply as these bullet points. They don't have to sound Confucian. They just need to be heartfelt. After you write such details down, try to answer these guide questions next:

- Do you eat when you experience extreme emotions from either end of the spectrum, for example, anger/sadness (on the negative end) or joy/excitement (on the positive end)?
- Do you eat in response to the same (or the same types of) people and situations?
- Do specific times and places cause you to think about food and/or eating?

When answered truthfully and thoughtfully, your responses to these questions can help you identify your triggers and confront them directly. It's a lot like putting a name to a face or vice versa. You gain power over something by being able to name it. It's factual; it's truthful. And truth is always liberating. Knowing your triggers—aka naming your nemeses—then leads to the next mile marker in your journey: **dealing with your specific triggers**.

Now that your triggers have names, you can take them on one by one. An important thing to do is to pinpoint their exact origin. Triggers are usually rooted in a past trauma or a painful memory but not always. Once triggers are … well … triggered, they can bring in a flood of images, sounds, tastes, etc., which are all part of the previous experience. They may be associated with things you'd rather forget, but now that they've been dredged up to the surface, you need to confront them and find a way to minimize or altogether remove their power over your life.

You may need a whole lot of courage and honesty to understand exactly how the past has gotten entangled in your present. Thankfully, it's not a herculean task. You just need time and a whole lot of patience to know and accept how food binges have become substitutes for something missing in your life. A dozen bantam bagels aren't your buffers against loneliness, but their bigger versions were what kept you company in the days following your parents' divorce. At some point, you have to realize that you were never alone. Despite the dissolution of their marriage, both your parents love you and have your back for life. The main point of this exercise is to weed out the lies and to cultivate the truths about yourself and your circumstances. You may sometimes need someone else's voice to clarify which is which, but that's exactly what the role of a support or care group is. You don't have to do it alone.

Many times, your triggers are nothing more than projections of your own inner turmoil. Your boss never said you were worthless, but you cast your own feeling of worthlessness onto her words and "hear" her say that nothing you do amounts to anything much. You're angry at your partner for ignoring your overt sexual advances and when they try to explain, you immediately shut down because their explanation sounds like they're angry at you, too. But really, the anger is a one-sided affair coming from your direction alone. In that case, it's fixable because it's well within your power to change.

Learn to draw the line between your feelings and thoughts versus those of others. You only need to be concerned and responsible for your own. This especially becomes important when you have to keep track of hyperarousal symptoms. Hyperarousal usually comes from posttraumatic stress disorder. Your body kicks into high gear as you remember your trauma and braces itself against some unseen assailant or impending doom. You may be watching the death of a beloved pet in a movie, but your body suddenly remembers you hunched over your golden retriever in his final moments as he crossed over the rainbow bridge. It remembers your shoulders shaking out huge sobs, the concrete pavement gritty and unyielding against your knees. The only thing that helped you survive that day was your best friend taking you out for a scrumptious dinner at your favorite Indian restaurant. And so, naan and butter chicken became your comfort food for every grief.

At some point, you need to start shifting away from food as your de facto comforter, satisfier, happiness generator, gap filler, Zen, Nirvana, etc. Keep your mind, heart, and body open to other coping mechanisms. When Forrest Gump's lifelong love, Jenny, left him after spending a night together, he goes off on a three-year run, crisscrossing the United States of America from coast to coast. When interviewed, he says he just felt like running. Mental health professionals know that it was because he was in serious pain —some might even call it depression. No one can survive the back-to-back losses of the two most important persons in their lives without acting out somehow.

Mentioning that story doesn't mean I'm telling you to become the next top ultramarathoner in the world. I'm simply saying that there are other and better ways to address your very needy emotions. Find those ones that will never make you feel guilty, embarrassed, condemned, and worse off than when you started. This also doesn't mean you give up on food as a comforter forever. It just means that you should never let it take the wheel away from you. You're the only one licensed to drive.

Dealing with your triggers can sometimes be as easy as stepping back and taking long, deep breaths. There are several breathing exercise tutorials online that can help you maximize all that oxygen flowing in and out of your lungs. The few minutes of inhaling and exhaling can clear your head enough for you to determine whether you're truly hungry or your emotions are the ones screaming for food. Even just five minutes of waiting before diving into a pile of bacon, eggs, and biscuits buys you time to check in with your feelings and make sure that they're not the ones forcing you to eat.

An ultimate goal of this book is not to teach you to hate food and eating. It's to help you embrace yourself and all your idiosyncrasies. Once you can accept every aspect of your being, it's likely that you can find other ways of dealing with your emotions. After all, you're not a flat, two-dimensional cartoon. Your identity can't and should never be reduced to "emotional eater" or "food binger". You're a multifaceted, complex person. You adore Freddie Mercury. You love your dog. You enjoy gardening. If you can constantly remind yourself that you're more than what you eat, you open yourself up to a whole spectrum of self-care methods to handle your emotions. Karaoke night to the songs of Queen? Forest walk with your Jack Russell? Build that long-pending vertical garden?

Layla was once an outdoor girl for all of her childhood and teen years, but things changed as she became a young adult, chained to a desk job as a copywriter in a top marketing agency. Within a year of starting work, she was overweight, suffering constantly from heartburns—no thanks to a constant fast-food spread laid out for overtiming staff, and no longer interested in hiking and camping. It depressed her to lose the fire that once got her going every day, so she ate some more whenever the realization hit her—and it seemed as though it did constantly every day.

Layla's friends and family were alarmed at her state. They gathered around her and encouraged her to seek help at a wellness center. She reluctantly agreed just to get them off her back. It was there where she met a counselor who was able to sift through her many issues and pinpoint exactly what was going on. She missed her dad, the hero of her life, who had lost a battle to cancer just before she graduated with a bachelor's degree. He was a burgers-fries-tacos kind of guy. Layla felt close to him when she ate his favorite foods. However, ironically, she shunned the outdoors because it was her dad's domain. There were too many reminders of how he laughed, how brave he was against the worst elements, and how much he loved his daughter.

As all this information came to light, Layla had the opportunity to evaluate her life thus far and what to do about her upside-down world. She slowly set things right by reducing her cravings for her dad's favorite foods and replaced them in her life with the thing that truly manifested her dad's love for her. Layla went back to spending more time in the mountains and forests to be closer to her dad again. It took several months, but she eventually left the food bingeing behind her and organized weekends away with family and friends to rekindle that wonderful pastime she shared with her favorite person in the whole wide world.

In Layla's case, many things worked in her favor: a strong support network, her own acceptance of needing help, and available and accessible wellness resources. Whether you have all or none of that, the important point to take away from her story is that she was able to overcome emotional eating only after she identified her triggers and got serious about dealing with them.

As I end this chapter and move on to the next, I encourage you to take time to fill in the worksheet below. I've described various scenarios that can happen to you. Your task is to complete the description with your own response to each scenario. Use your gut reac-

CONQUER EMOTIONAL EATING | 85

tion. Sorry, no multiple choice for you; your trigger/s is/are your very own, no one else's.

Scenario One:

You hit the jackpot at a slot machine in a Las Vegas casino. What do you do immediately after collecting your winnings? _____

How does your reaction rate in light of everything that you've read in the book so far? _____

Do you need to change your reaction? Explain. _____

Scenario Two:

You rear-ended the vehicle in front of you, causing major damage to your car and the other one. What do you do as soon as you get home? _____

How does your reaction rate in light of everything that you've read in the book so far? _____

Do you need to change your reaction? Explain. _____

Scenario Three:

You're home alone on a Friday night, too tired and broke to go out with friends. How do you spend the evening by yourself? _____

How does your reaction rate in light of everything that you've read in the book so far? _____

Do you need to change your reaction? Explain. _____

Scenario Four:

You've just seen a piece of paper with the name of your partner's ex and a phone number in their trouser pocket. They're away for the weekend and you have no way of reaching them to ask about it. What do you do while waiting for their return? _____

How does your reaction rate in light of everything that you've read in the book so far? _____

Do you need to change your reaction? Explain. _____

Scenario Five:

You're sitting at your kitchen table full of end-month bills, screaming for your attention. Your work hours had just been cut in half, so you're worried about your finances. What do you do? _____

How does your reaction rate in light of everything that you've read in the book so far? _____

Do you need to change your reaction? Explain. _____

Scenario Six:

You failed to reach your quarterly quota at work and your fairly decent boss expressed disappointment at your shortfall. What do you do when you leave the office for the day? _____

How does your reaction rate in light of everything that you've read in the book so far? _____

Do you need to change your reaction? Explain. _____

The force ... er ... connection between your triggers and emotions can be quite strong. Once you trip a trigger, your emotions immediately come to the surface. Since they were awoken rather unceremoniously—complete with bedhead and wrinkled PJs—they're usually foul and ready to push you to do your worst. You don't want that to happen, of course, so the upcoming chapter can help you sort them out, understand why they happen, and figure out a way to break the chain reaction from trigger to (mostly negative) emotions to unpleasant eating behaviors.

5

TUNE IN TO YOUR EMOTIONS

Michaela's husband arrived home late one night and immediately served her with divorce papers. He yelled that he had gotten tired of their marriage and didn't want to have anything to do with her anymore. "You're no longer the woman I married three years ago," he said. "You look like a blimp." For a couple of years after that abrupt ending, Michaela leaned heavily on tubs of ice cream, gallons of iced tea, and XL bags of potato chips to buoy up her spirits. She was so devastated by her ex's harsh comment about her weight gain, that she piled on some more pounds to dull the humiliation, guilt, and shame she felt. She never even questioned her former hubby's snide remark. Like the literary scarlet letter, she wore the word "blimp" on her chest and it was a ton of bricks that dragged her down to exhaustion every day.

It wasn't until she went shopping for her daughter's school clothes that Michaela finally woke up from her stupor. Somebody complimented her for her "granddaughter's" cute outfits and it was a hard slap on her face. She got a good look at herself in a fitting room mirror and realized how old she appeared, so much older than her actual age. She had to pump the brakes on her downward spiral.

With the help of her inner circle of family and friends and a professional, one of the first things Michaela learned to do was to listen to her emotions. She had unconsciously tuned them out that fateful night and packed them away somewhere near the back wall of her closet. It was time to air them out and process them for her healing and recovery to begin. By dealing with her emotions first, she realized—among many, many things —how much love there was between her daughter and her, and that was all that mattered at that point. Instead of moping around the house, agonizing over her ex's departure, and neglecting her child, she discovered activities that she and her little one could do together, including playdates with her daughter's friends. There she met other moms who invited her for this fun run and that Zumba class. Before long, Michaela was able to gain more friends and decrease the alone time she had in close proximity to her kitchen. Michaela's struggle with emotional eating became much more manageable, when she began focusing on her emotions first, understanding their nature and origin, and finding alternative and better ways of taking care of them.

This may be somebody else's story and not your own, but it presents a few points worth mulling over. Emotions are an important part of being human, so accept them. They make you, you. They're not like cancer that you have to or can gouge out of your life. You just need to know how to live with them. To learn to live with them, you have to be willing to look them straight in the eye and say, "I see you. You are a part of me. You are mine."

Emotional eating doesn't happen because you can't say no to food. As many as there are Michaelas in the world, who indulge in potato chips, iced tea, and ice cream to push away their pain, there are plenty more who eat the same fare without obsessing about them. They eat the "comfort food" and then move on. End of story. So, it's not about saying yes or no to food and having power (or no power) over them. It's about exercising power over your emotions. It's not called emotional eating for nothing. In the phrase, emotions come first syntactically and—more importantly—conceptually. The so-called triggers I discussed in the previous chapter aren't connected to food; they're linked to emotions. And vice versa. It's not the food's fault.

In a sense, food is like a victim here. It gets such a bad rap for causing ill health and overly burdened bathroom scales, but it's just a poor scapegoat that can't even defend itself against its accusers. Yes, it's absolutely delicious when laden with sugars, herbs, spices, fats, and just the right amount of salt, and plenty of people run to it for its many sensory delights to the eyes, tongue, and nose. But food never designated itself an emotional crutch. It wasn't even born that way nor did it volunteer to be so. If anything, it was some rather devious human being who started calling it that and the label stuck.

Food does produce, enhance, or modify certain hormones and chemicals in your body; I had mentioned dopamine in an earlier section of this book. It gives you that happy, feel-good effect as you chow down on that barbecued chicken leg. Other hormones that can be affected by your food intake (or lack of it) are endorphins, oxytocin, and serotonin. With a simple tweak to the amount, frequency, and quality of food you ingest (plus other things like sleep, exercise, etc.), these hormones can serve you well or make your life a living hell. But food per se is just there to nourish you, keep you strong and alert, and energize you. It may give you a lot of pleasurable feels, too, but that is not food's main function. Its role as an emotional crutch—when you depend on it primarily or ... yikes ... solely to make you happy and scare the blues away, among many of your other emotional needs—is an artificial construct. We, humans, made it to be so the first time one of us put all our faith in its efficacy to bring comfort and relief—even if temporarily—in the midst of our struggles.

The use of food as an emotional crutch is sometimes subtle and even goes unnoticed. A poet friend must have at least seven mugs of black coffee every day or she can't string together a verse even in a life-and-death situation. The frazzled homemaker waits for the clock to strike four p.m. and off she goes to the kitchen to pour herself a glass of wine and spread a charcuterie board for her own version of happy hour. A commercial truck driver needs to have Twizzlers on him at all times to stay awake during the long, lonely stretches of empty highways he drives on at midnight.

However, not every instance of food as an emotional crutch is bad or an indicator of some deeper problems. Despite your seeming dependence on KitKat to fuel you every two hours, it doesn't interfere with the normal flow of your thoughts and emotions. When your partner forgets your birthday, you don't hide in the bathroom to eat a whole mango cake by yourself. Instead, you give them hell and give it a few minutes or an hour at most before you get together again and "make up for lost time".

Before your use of food as an emotional crutch takes a turn for the worse, stand in your kitchen and address all the edible contents of your cupboards, shelves, pantry, fridge, and freezer: "You are not my emotional crutch. You are not the master of me. I have complete control over myself and my emotions." And then turn and walk away. You may or may not follow the suggestion literally—depends on what kind of humor you have. The point is this: one day (soon, I hope), you need to draw the line and remove the crutch from underneath you. Food and eating are so much more than a crutch. And you have so much more than them to get you through your emotional turmoil.

You can change your view of food and eating as an emotional crutch by reminding yourself of their true place in your life. When you eat, you do so because your body needs replenishment for expended energy. You eat because you want to provide all your organs with the necessary nutrients to keep them running and you, living. You eat because your body is genuinely hungry and not because you have nothing else to do at the moment.

Of course, a good pep talk to yourself is one thing; transformative actions are another. You can begin by eating and savoring every mouthful. Chew slowly; learn from the bovines, who never look rushed while rolling the cud around in their mouth. Don't shovel food into your maw. Use human-sized cutlery that measures out human-sized bite pieces. Alternate between drinking water and eating. Don't eat while trying to beat a project deadline or watching *The Crown* on Netflix. Let eating be a stand-alone activity, not to be done at the same time as scrolling through Instagram or doing a weekend *World of Warcraft* marathon. Sure, have some bistro music playing in the background for a suitable ambiance, but nothing that will get you up and jumping or hunched over in a good cry. Bring back eating to its original form as a basic and essential human function, beneficial to your body but not a buttress for your emotions.

Whenever food comes to mind, don't switch to autopilot and eat straightaway. Press pause and walk through the process of removing the crutch. Rather than asking yourself a series of questions—who has time to have that questionnaire readily available every time a craving hits—just don't. Don't eat. I don't mean completely ignore the hunger and starve yourself the whole day. If it's a genuine hunger, you should actually be able to delay it. Emotional hunger stridently demands that you feed yourself pronto. Physical hunger can be postponed. In an earlier chapter, I discussed their differences at length. You should keep that knowledge in mind when emotional hunger tries to trick you.

Instead of immediately feeding yourself, do something else. Stretch. Walk around the garden. Play fetch with the dog. Go look for that thing in your glove compartment that's been bothering you for some time now, even though you can't remember why. Once you've created that space between you and the hunger, do a deep dive and dissect it. Once you're fairly certain that it's not the physical kind, see if you can discover the real root of the craving. What's going on with you? Are you mad at your neighbor who "accidentally" pruned your rosebushes again? Are you stressed about being laid off? Are you worried about your partner being out on a "work" trip?

If you have time to journal about it, do so right then and there. Or if you're constrained by time, take down some bullet points about your hunger and write them into your journal later. You can then review them for a deeper understanding of the emotions involved, but for now, you just need to do a quick look-see to determine if food is really to answer. Is it related to the quality of the day you're currently having? Or maybe the week unfolding badly for you? How about that time of month? No, that question isn't just for women as men can also worry about bills at a set date every month, like clockwork.

As soon as you've pinpointed the root, see if you can satisfy the real cause in a timely manner with the correct solution. Walk the trail around the lake nearby for a breather from all the busyness of life. Have a sit-down with your partner about your relationship issues. Talk to your boss about some extraordinary challenges you have at work. Call your mom in post-surgery recovery at the hospital to know how she's doing. Sometimes, these little adjustments to your day are all you need to prevent emotional eating from taking over your life.

However, not every instance of emotional eating can be solved by a tiny tweak to your schedule and plans. Some of them are not just about "this very moment". Your extreme anguish over a recent breakup isn't just about losing that particular partner. It's about a lifetime of people rejecting you for not being "good enough". In such cases, batten down. You may be in for a long, arduous process of reckoning and recovery. Definitely, you shouldn't try to do it alone. Seek professional help or surround yourself with people you can trust with your life. Keep yourself accountable to them. They'll have your best interest at heart and will have your back until you find your way back from that pit you've fallen into.

Whenever the fake hunger, aka emotional hunger, strikes, be ready with an activity or activities that will steer you away from that siren song of sorts. Have at least three to five things to do, readily available and doable in your back pocket. Being prepared this way means that emotional hunger can never ever get the best of you or catch you off guard. Your vulnerable parts are safely behind the armor of alternative activities.

Even while you restore food and eating into their rightful and true roles and functions in your life, it's also time to deal with your emotions and face them squarely. Let's go back to your journal. If you've done your "assignment" and been honest in describing your thoughts, emotions, situational details, actions, reactions, etc., on its pages, then you have in your hands a

CONQUER EMOTIONAL EATING | 99

valuable tool for unlocking your freedom from emotional eating.

When it comes to writing about your emotions, approach the task in the same way you approach writing about eating—with curiosity, not judgement; with a determination to learn, not a resolve to condemn. Your notebook becomes forensic evidence in helping you sort out what's happening with your demeanor. Mindfully noting down your emotions and the details surrounding them fixes your attention at the right place. The worst thing you can do is ignore or avoid your emotions. Learn from Michaela who tuned hers out for a couple of years.

Just because you deny the existence of your emotions doesn't mean that they'll work things out by themselves. You need to own them; after all, they belong to you. When you sweep your emotions under the rug, you're saying that they're not valid and they don't warrant your precious time. By extension, you're also saying that you're not valid. You shouldn't pay any mind to your emotions because they're bothersome. You really shouldn't be allowed any emotions.

Your emotions are a part of the whole you. Without them, you're less than a human being. They're what set us apart from robots. People feel; automatons don't. The "scary" bit about a film like *Blade Runner* (both iterations) is that robots have started having feels and independently coherent thoughts. You, on the other hand, are going in the opposite direction, wanting to achieve robot characteristics with the denial of your emotions.

When you turn your head away from your emotions, you're communicating to yourself that you don't deserve to be a Homo sapiens. That immediately puts you on the wrong side of science, religion, and your Aunt Gracie from two blocks away. You're allowed to feel feelings, you know? Also, when you don't face your emotions, you lose the opportunity to grow as a person. The Greek philosopher, Socrates, supposedly said, "An unexamined life is not worth living." If you don't give yourself time to reflect upon your life—examine it, if you will—and everything that's a part of it (read: your emotions), then you come out of that moment with zero growth. You learn nothing about yourself; you learn nothing about your place in the world. How do you expect to do better next time if you've not identified your areas that need improvement? How do you know which emotions are at play and require attention, if you don't scrutinize them? Don't you immediately check on that knocking sound under the hood of your car? Acknowledging your emotions is doing exactly that: stopping, popping open the hood, and inspecting the source of the noise. You want to make sure that things don't escalate and become a $5,000 expense at the workshop.

Emotions don't just affect your mind and figurative heart. They're also capable of inducing physiological responses, some of which can lead to the literal death of a person. Nowadays, we know that "broken heart" is not just a poetic phrase; it can be an actual tearing of the cardio muscles, provoked by a situation of unexpected and severe stress.

You may be afraid of facing your emotions because you were brought up to shun "making a scene". Rather than coming at your cheating boyfriend with arms swinging, you opt to seethe in your bedroom until a TV ad entices you to order something via DoorDash. You have to remember that a passive-aggressive silence and screaming at the top of your lungs are not your only means of handling your emotions. Those two are at opposite ends of the response spectrum. Have you had a look at what lies in the middle? Acquaint yourself with the middle ground. It exists and it's available for you to explore and use.

To understand emotions further, let's borrow some knowledge from everybody's favorite Pixar "emotion" picture, *Inside Out*. When you express emotions, they're never just one-layered. Several emotions come into play all at the same time, but others have bigger "voices" than the rest for that particular situation. They're the ones you hear most clearly because they dominate the scene. However, the background action doesn't stop. Other emotions are still lurking nearby, finding a way to gain the upper hand. Someone grabs a megaphone; another stands on a ladder. A third emotion tries to float by on a balloon. With all that activity initiated by a single trigger, what you're really dealing with here is not a monolithic anger or a monolithic fear. It's multiple multifaceted, multi-layered emotions. To deal with all of them at the same time, you need a system, a mechanism, or a structure that can manage the load of several individual emotions coming together in a complex whole. More about that shortly.

We humans supposedly developed emotions as a means of discovering our place and way around the world. As our ancestors processed information with their senses, they were either drawn to it or not, depending on the kind of response the information evoked. Those responses were our original emotions. If we are to believe the Gary Larson cartoon (*The Far Side*) of a prehistoric man running away from a flame-filled cave mouth, the discovery of fire must have caused one helluva fright to the oversized muscle bag to trigger his flight.

The caveman's response to fire was of the negative kind. It probably made him feel uncomfortable to stand too close to something hot, making him sweat under the animal pelts he wore. He must have even touched a burning piece of wood, causing him to feel pain on his hand. All that made him perceive a threat to his existence, so he moved his body away from the cause of his responses. His act of escaping is one of the main behaviors motivated by negative emotions. Emotions such as anger, apprehension, fear, guilt, jealousy, pain, revulsion, sadness, etc., make you want to remove yourself from the danger. Or you might just want to walk things back a bit, you know, de-escalate the stress. Either way, negative emotions compel you to avoid the same scenario or thing, or person the next time or find ways to control it.

On the other hand, positive emotions attract you toward the world. This is the neighborhood of excitement, happiness, joy, etc. These emotions give you pleasure and are created when you observe that your needs as a human being are met within the environment you're in. For example, let's go back to the little caveman's moment of discovering fire. While it may have initially led him to run away, he did eventually come back. Upon his return—lo and behold!—he learned that the fire that made him scamper away was also the same fire that could make his slab of bison meat tastier. It didn't take long for his friends and him to figure out other ways to use the pile of heat and light. They had such an overwhelming sense of contentment that they began stamping their feet and mimicking the movement of animals and tree branches. And that was how the first rave was organized: a group of happy people making their own music and dancing to their own beat, in the brightness of light they created themselves.

Beyond a definition of emotions according to evolution, emotions are those intangible things inside us that help us make sense of the world. They emerge from within us, so we can understand experiences and relationships in relation to ourselves. They also help us identify the necessities for our existence. As a very young child still unexposed to harsh realities in the world, your puppy dies and you don't quite know what to make of it. Then you start feeling a tightness in your chest, your shoulders heave, and then something liquid forms in your eyes. Before long, your folks fuss over you. You hear them exclaim, "Oh no! You're crying," and you figure out they're talking about you and what's happening with you. Soon, your mom comes up to you and asks, "Honey, are you sad?" In your short conversation with her, it's then that you figure out exactly what she meant by her question. This event involving the loss of something, someone precious is what everyone calls death and your chest tightening is the appropriate reaction to it. They call your experience grief. When there's a lack of one-to-one correspondence between event and emotional response, that's when professionals start digging into potential psychological conditions plaguing you.

Paul Gilbert (2009), a renowned British clinical psychologist, lists three distinct emotional systems responsible for handling your emotions. One is called the Safety System. The job description is in its name. It's in charge of, say, kicking in your fight-or-flight response to keep you safe. It processes your simultaneously felt anger and fear at a driver weaving in and out of traffic to (a) call 911 to report the unfolding, dangerous traffic violation, (b) pull to the side of the interstate when highway patrol comes speeding past to chase the offender down, and (c) double-check that your kids are safely strapped in their car seats. It helps you calculate if running into a burning barn to save cattle and poultry in the middle of nowhere is worth it or not. The Safety System is likely to rein in your impulse and make you think multiple times before attempting a foolhardy feat.

The Drive System is probably the achiever's dominant mechanism. It harnesses your younger sister's love and joy at doing math and keeps her motivated to qualify for the International Math Olympiad. The system allows you to derive pleasure and happiness from attaining a sought-after goal. With this system at work, your life trajectory seems to go nowhere but up, up, and up! And that is also the system's flaw. When you don't achieve your target, the sense of failure is palpable and weighs heavily on your shoulders.

The remainder in the trio of emotional systems is the Soothing System. It's all about drawing contentment from your relationships with other people. You may find its roots in your childhood when you customarily begin to experience the love and devotion of people in your life. If you were never the recipient of such in your early years, this system can be quite inutile—or even downright non-existent—in helping you cope with distress and anxiety.

Emotions need one, two, or all three systems together to be fully under your control at any given moment. Of course, you and I wish that life were fair and every person on earth has their emotional systems in perfect working order. Sadly, this isn't the case. In the absence or lackluster operation of your emotional systems, you inadvertently turn to food to make up for their short-coming. Or you probably never even knew that such systems existed inside you, so you cast about for different solutions, aka food, to take care of your emotions.

As you should be able to tell by now, food can be quite the trickster. It can imitate the output of your emotional systems, but it can never take their place. It's like asking Alexa to set your grandpa's wind-up alarm clock to go off at six a.m. It's quaint to think that Alexa can suddenly grow hands to fulfill that command, but it ain't gonna happen. At best, it can remind you to set it yourself because you're the one with arms, hands, and fingers. Food can offer your body so many other benefits to keep it healthy and strong, but it can't cross the divide and do the same thing for your emotions. It wasn't created for them. It can only pretend to do so and the result can leave you in a worse state than before.

At this point, the best thing you can do for your emotions is to sit with them and get to know them. I hesitate to use "get in touch with your emotions" because some people may react differently and agitatedly to it. When you say that to men (and even women) brought up under difficult circumstances and/or belonging to a much older generation, they can look at you askance, hackles raised, feeling insulted that you should insinuate something about their toughness (or lack of it) or their ability to survive under harsh conditions. And really, they don't have time for your touchy-feely exercises. Therein lies a probable reason for many individuals falling into emotional eating.

If you were never given the opportunity to get acquainted with your emotions, especially by the adults responsible for you in your formative years, then you lost an opportunity to develop that facet of your being. The good news is that it's not too late to catch up. You can still know your emotions and how to deal with them at this stage in your life.

You can begin by naming the emotion you're experiencing at the moment. Giving something a name gives you power over it, as I had said much earlier in this book. This principle is true across all studies and disciplines, from anthropology to zoology. The singular name makes it easier for you to talk about it at length. Imagine saying "that thing that you use to open a lock" instead of just "key". You'd be out of breath before you could get the actual point across. Earlier, I had called the exercise "naming your nemeses", but I do acknowledge that not all emotions are to be treated as annoyances. There are some emotions, belonging to the positive side of the spectrum, which should also be identified, so you can relish them for the good that they bring into your life.

If you struggle with what to call an emotion, the University of New Hampshire created two tools that can find you the right name. The first tool is simply called an Emotions Table. It's structured like any standard table of nomenclature (a system of naming things). Each column is topped with a general term in boldface and all caps. If some of them are unfamiliar to you, feel free to pick up a dictionary and check their meaning. (No shame in getting a little help from friends.) The general term is followed by a few second-level terms in all caps and then third-level ones in initial caps, altogether leading you deep into the territory of specifics.

Emotions Table:

SURPRISE	FEAR	ANGER	DISGUST	SAD	HAPPY
• STARTLED	• HUMILIATED	• HURT	• DISAPPROVAL	• GUILTY	• OPTIMISTIC
○ Shocked	○ Disrespected	○ Devastated	○ Judgmental	○ Remorseful	○ Inspired
○ Dismayed	○ Ridiculed	○ Embarrassed	○ Loathing	○ Ashamed	○ Open
• CONFUSED	• REJECTED	• THREATENED	• DISAPPOINTED	• ABANDONED	• INTIMATE
○ Disillusioned	○ Alienated	○ Jealous	○ Repugnant	○ Ignored	○ Playful
○ Perplexed	○ Inadequate	○ Insecure	○ Revolted	○ Victimized	○ Sensitive
• AMAZED	• SUBMISSIVE	• HATEFUL	• AWFUL	• DESPAIR	• PEACEFUL
○ Astonished	○ Insignificant	○ Violated	○ Revulsion	○ Powerless	○ Hopeful
○ Awe	○ Worthless	○ Resentful	○ Detestable	○ Vulnerable	○ Loving
• EXCITED	• INSECURE	• MAD	• AVOIDANCE	• DEPRESSED	• POWERFUL
○ Eager	○ Inferior	○ Enraged	○ Aversion	○ Inferior	○ Provocative
○ Energetic	○ Inadequate	○ Furious	○ Hesitant	○ Empty	○ Courageous

	FEAR	ANGER		SAD	HAPPY
	• ANXIOUS	• AGGRESSIVE		• LONELY	• ACCEPTED
	○ Worried	○ Provoked		○ Abandoned	○ Respected
	○ Overwhelmed	○ Hostile		○ Isolated	○ Fulfilled
	• SCARED	• FRUSTRATED		• BORED	• PROUD
	○ Frightened	○ Infuriated		○ Apathetic	○ Important
	○ Terrified	○ Irritated		○ Indifferent	○ Confident
		• DISTANT			• INTERESTED
		○ Withdrawn			○ Amused
		○ Suspicious			○ Inquisitive
		• CRITICAL			• JOYFUL
		○ Skeptical			○ Liberated
		○ Sarcastic			○ Ecstatic

The Emotions Wheel is similar to the first tool except for the shape. You begin your search for the right term from the center of the wheel. You then work outward toward the most specific word you can find. You can use your bodily "data" to inform your options. Is your heart racing? Are you sweating profusely? Are you having difficulty swallowing? Is your carotid artery throbbing? Are you able to get a full night's sleep?

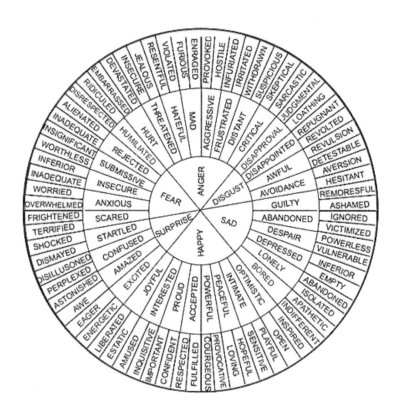

Your responses to these kinds of questions weed out several choices because the sign or symptom you're experiencing can apply only to one or a few and not all terms listed on the wheel. Ultimately, you are left with THE one correct name for your emotion.

However, as the movie, *Inside Out*, showed us, remember that you may actually be experiencing more than one emotion at the same time, making it difficult for you to pick one. That's okay and expected. You're allowed to pick five different emotions, knowing that each is valid as far as your current experience is concerned. As with writing down your emotions, don't be a Judge Judy to yourself when it comes to naming the emotion and experiencing it fully. Accept the good, bad, and ugly that you stumble upon. Saying that you're "raging against God" because you can't accept the loss of your cancer-stricken partner is more authentic than "yes, I'm happy that they're in a better place now". Your emotions are in turmoil. Call them what they are, so you don't end up hiding behind a bucket of buffalo wings. Working head-on with facts in an era of fake news is important and refreshing. That's where and when true change happens.

Managing your emotions may entail you scheduling time for them. When you don't do that deliberately, you may end up having unwanted visitors knocking at your door at the most inappropriate time. They're like your dreaded in-laws. They've been telling you to invite them to your home, but you've been finding every excuse under the sun to keep them away. Finally, they show up at midnight to surprise you, just when you and your partner are about to do vigorous, happy things together.

Set a regular time to check in with your emotions. If you can offer tea and sympathy to other people, you can do the same for yourself. Review your journal. See if there are some items in there that you may need to take up with your emotions. Listen to what they're telling you. Are there some things about your life you need to change? Is there someone you need to speak with to sort out a hidden resentment at them? Ruminate. Reflect. For the religiously inclined, this is when you pray and meditate. Above anything else, be kind to your emotions, which is code for "be kind to yourself". Don't be afraid to give yourself the best ugly cry that you can manage—with snot all over your face. There are people who find a secluded spot in a forest to let out a primal scream. Whatever works for you, find a way to release your pent-up emotions. It's no coincidence that several businesses have opened up, offering people safe ways to vent. You can break plates, throw knives at targets, or smash walls with a mallet, all under the watchful gaze of safety coordinators. And once you're done with all that, come back to the land of the living. It'll all be okay. You won't even need a dozen donuts to know that to be true.

Before we move on to the next chapter, I encourage you to do this short exercise, which I'll call, "The Favourite Food Mental Map". Think of your favorite food (veggie pizza for me, just as an example for doing this exercise). Write it down on a clean sheet of paper and draw a box around it. Next, list some of the reasons why you like it. Spread the words/phrases around the name of your favorite food. (For me, it could be three things: I love Italian cuisine; I love vegetables; I love lots of cheese.) Draw boxes around each answer and connect the individual box to your favorite food box. Under each reason, probe further by reflecting upon why it's significant. (For example, I love vegetable pizza because I love Italian food. I love Italian food because my paternal grandmother was Italian and she always kneaded the best pizza dough for us every day. I'm thinking about veggie pizza now because I miss my grandma, whose death anniversary is today.)

Your map may be narrower or broader than mine, but the objective of the exercise is this: to equip you with a tool for understanding how specific foods relate to your emotions and vice versa. You don't have to do a whole bunch of maps right now, but when you're spending time with your emotions, this can be one of those things for helping you know yourself.

May your map help you navigate your way out of emotional eating into a newfound freedom and power over food.

6

GIVE IN TO YOUR REAL NEEDS

You're more than halfway through this book now. It should be abundantly clear already that food is good and beneficial. It's not the devil incarnate that makes you bloat up like a bullfrog and feel guilty about it after. However, it's not what you should reach out for when your emotions are being needy. Attention-seeking emotions require emotional solutions, not food meant for the physical body. In light of recent times, that's like giving antibiotics to a person with a viral infection. Antibiotics are for fighting bacteria; antiviral drugs and vaccines are for countering viruses. They don't, can't, and shouldn't cross over.

The more you spend time knowing your emotions, the more you realize that what you really require is not something that food can ever fully satisfy in you. It might feel that way for a hot minute, but that satiation fades away quickly and you're left with an even bigger hole to fill than before. What you should be looking for are long-term answers, aka the fulfillment of your real needs.

Close to the mid-20th century, Abraham Maslow, a renowned American psychologist, came up with a pyramid-shaped diagram, detailing the fundamental needs of human beings. The base is made up of physiological needs: food, water, sleep, sex, breath, etc. The second level is composed of matters that give humans a sense of security: employment, wealth, health, etc. The third has everything to do with a sense of belonging, e.g., different kinds of relationships. The penultimate level is all about a human's sense of worth: confidence, two-way respect, achievement, etc. The fifth and final level involves a human's self-actualization, so the needs listed under this include morality, creativity, etc.—the pinnacle of being human and not any other creature.

From the time it was presented until today, there's been a lot of discussion about Maslow's model. As with any academic concept, it has a group that agrees with it and another that opposes it. However, that's not the point of why I mention it here. What is important to see is that it's a well-established fact that humans have needs that define our thoughts, emotions, actions, and words. Our needs are a part of what makes us human. Their absence can make you a rather questionable human being—how can you call yourself one if you don't have any needs?

Tony Robbins, a respected American life coach, author, speaker, and philanthropist, riffed on Maslow's needs pyramid to create his own set of six human needs, which must be attended to every day:

1. You need **certainty**. You want no drama and grief (that is, pain) in your life. You aim for your existence to coast as smoothly as a billionaire's yacht on the tranquil blue waters of the Sargasso Sea. You're hardwired to seek pleasure, so all your engagements, decisions, and goals are focused on achieving it. As both pain and pleasure are a part of your time on Earth, you can't escape either. The secret to living with both and still attaining certainty is choosing in such a way that pain runs only for a short time while pleasure goes on track for the long term. You don't want to mix that up so that pain does the marathon, while pleasure only does the sprint.

2. The complex human that you are must also have **uncertainty** or **variety** to keep balanced and be better grounded. An unvarying situation

doesn't leave you with room for growth. It might as well be a flatline state you're living in if you don't allow for a bit of spice and zest into your life. You want appropriate doses of excitement as stimuli for keeping you engaged and vested in your continued existence.

3. You require **significance** as a person. You need to know that you matter and that the things you do, say, or think count for something valuable in this world. Even when you just yawn, it should cause a sunflower variety in Africa to grow taller and more golden as evidence that you're not just a flash in the pan.

4. You need **love** and **connection**. There's no escaping the fact that you are a social being. Even if you may be independent and self-sufficient, you still need an extra pair of hands to carry the brand-new grand piano up to your fifth-floor apartment. You still need a shoulder to cry on when you're having the feels. Watch *I Am Legend* and understand why Dr. Robert Neville required a dog to keep him company and a comatose zombie vampire to talk to because it'll show you that it is utterly human to seek relationships of any kind—even in the midst of an apocalypse and you're the last person standing.

5. You have to have **growth**. Imagine life without room for you to develop from childhood to adulthood—and that's not just in reference to your physical body. Growth must also happen for your mind, emotions, and spirit as well. Professionals (biologists, medical doctors, psychologists, etc.) recognize that many forms of stunting can be problematic as they prevent you from reaching your ultimate personhood. Besides bonsai, I can't think of any other growthless state as wonderful and welcome. You are expected to grow and must grow.

6. You need to produce or perform a **contribution** that makes the world a better place than when you first arrived in it. You desire to leave some sort of a legacy that says you were here and you did good. It's like your initials carved on the bark of a tree for future generations to admire and remember you by. It may not always be as impactful as you want it to be, but you can tell yourself that you tried. One dollar to a total stranger of a hobo, for coffee, is still one dollar.

Robbins makes a distinction for the last two needs (growth and contribution) by describing them as "needs of the soul", which can only be realized if the first four (certainty, variety, significance, and connection) are addressed initially. Soul requirements cannot precede the basic four. There's an almost linear direction to follow in the Robbins version of human needs.

As with so many things in this world, each need can be met through more than one means—or as the old saying goes, "There's more than one way to skin a cat." My earlier illustration of the fictional Dr. Neville captures that idea. You can have a semblance of a connection from either a pet, a terrifying virus carrier, or a photograph of a lost love. You can also have an experience of certainty from reading a book, shooting up on an illegal substance, or eating a tomahawk steak solo. These examples are either good, bad, or neutral, depending on their final outcome in your life. By extension, eating in and of itself isn't a bad thing to give you a measure of certainty, but if it comes into the picture as anything other than a fulfillment of a physical requirement, then that's when you may need to reconsider its role in your existence.

And here's another matter to bear in mind when meeting your needs: don't have just one object be the end-all and be-all of half of your needs. Or don't let a single behavior be the means of attaining three of the six needs listed. Don't let a giant tray of Ferrero Rocher eaten in one sitting be your source of certainty, variety, and significance altogether. Just imagine how disastrous that scenario can become when you need to give it up for your own good. You won't even be able to see the good beyond it anymore because the power of the chocolate is simply too overwhelming. You're not supposed to give anyone, anything, or any place that kind of control over you.

Your real needs are explicit. Unless you're playing the denial game with them or being deliberately obtuse to yourself and your situation, they are obvious and make their demands very clear. In such a setup, you should be ready to answer them directly and concisely. No point beating around the bush or finding alternative solutions. If you're completely exhausted from a long day at the office, you have no business lingering in the kitchen and poking around in the pantry. As soon as you've had a proper dinner, take a hot shower and go straight to bed. Do not pass go. Do not collect a whole bag of Oreos and take to your bedside table.

When you're bored, don't remain in your house. Walk to the nearest park and feed some chopped lettuce to the pond ducks. Sign up for some random free class at the Y. You're never too old or too young to learn something new. When you're missing your family a few hundred miles away, volunteer at an animal shelter and play with their residents. If you're not clear about your real need, you should always make time and space to listen to your body, mind, heart, and spirit to know what it is and not make the mistake of cooking and eating a dozen pancakes at three in the morning.

I've mentioned in an earlier section or two of the book that there's a one-to-one correspondence between your need and its fulfiller. Do yourself a favor and just go right ahead and give your need the one thing that quiets it down. If your stomach is actually hungry, give it food. If you're mortified because your partner left you for your best friend, cry about it, but don't let Ben & Jerry's anywhere near you. If the pain of a breakup is too unbearable, seek a professional listener, aka a therapist.

When you're addressing emotional eating, the last thing you want to pile on your plate is a bunch of dos and don'ts to regulate your behavior. You don't suffer from a lack of self-control, remember? Instead, get real with your emotions and stop judging yourself. I'm now close to the end of this book, so I won't repeat myself by outlining once again exactly how you should deal with your emotions. If need be, backtrack to the earlier chapters yourself and reread the important pointers for addressing them. The important thing is that you don't make the mistake of using food and eating as the solutions. Ever. Again.

If you don't know what to do specifically or where to start in your journey away from emotional eating, then try a bit of meditation. It's a safe space and moment for you to be still and get in touch with your emotions. There are multiple online resources to tap into for free meditation guides. Don't forget to use the keywords "meditation, mindful, eating" to get what you need.

If meditation doesn't cut it for you because it's too esoteric or ambiguous for your needs, then use the following suggestions:

- Take a rest break when you're all wound up and on edge. As any experienced person knows, if you keep winding up that old-school clock, you will break its spring and render it useless— possibly forever. Same principle applies to you when you push yourself to the brink of a breakdown. You have got to stop and press pause before you teeter over the edge into oblivion.
- Participate in activities that require your full attention if you want to "empty" your mind. Go to a museum and sketch a sculpture. Learn how to do the salsa. Hit the bunny slope on your first attempt to snowboard. These kinds of proactive activities leave no room for the devil

to set up a workshop in your mind—to counter an old saying.

- Adjust your expectations when you're neither here nor there with your energy levels. Understand that it's okay if you're sometimes not operating at full capacity. A season of blahs happens to all of us from time to time. You don't always have to be switched on, so don't be judgemental of yourself when you miss the mark a time or two.

- Watch a Monty Python comedy or any funny film when you're in despair. Again, despair is nothing to be ashamed of as a part of life. Find something to do that allows you to see that your despair is not the end of the world. I have read some stories of people volunteering at soup kitchens or hospices to help them shift their point of view and appreciate what they already have. It can sometimes be a bit patronizing of them to say so, but if you can channel that realization into something that truly benefits a community with no strings attached, then you're doing the right thing of turning your despair into a beneficial outcome.

- Do. Your. Homework. Now. Don't stick your head into the fridge and look for something to bite, nibble, sip, or gulp. Get with the schedule.

Remind yourself that there's no taking back the minutes and hours that pass as you delay your work. Once the time is gone, it's gone for good. You are not in possession of Hermione Granger's time-turner.

- Find a quiet corner and sit still when stress is drowning you. Practice some breathing exercises. There are plenty of video tutorials online to choose from. Take as much time as needed to get to a place when things are peaceful inside you again.

- Call or text a loved one when you're feeling blue. That kind of burden is not meant to be carried alone. You don't have any excuse not to connect at a time when there is an abundance of social media platforms. A free, steady, reliable, and readily available video call is no longer sci-fi mumbo-jumbo. With one tap of a phone app icon, you can watch your baby take their first steps. Or observe the wedding of your best friend on the other side of the world.

- Tidy up your room if you need some mental clarity. The literal clean-up sometimes translates to a mental clear-up as you allow your mind to move away from its primary stressors into a zero-stress situation. A stress-free zone is completely unrelated to environments you associate with a pressure cooker. There's no escalation of activity or pace. It's just all flat, steady, and predictable. That's the perfect breather for you to take. Come back in only when you know you're completely ready.

- Make a list to anchor your thoughts and emotions. It can be a bucket list of new travel destinations to visit or a gratefulness roster of things you appreciate in your life. Or any list that requires a moment of slowing down and reflecting. The time it takes for you to note items is time to keep your thinking and emoting from darting every which way like a skittish colt in a corral.
- Go the primal way and scream into a pillow or rip a classic yellow pages directory to pieces. It's a way of expending all your energies until you have nothing left to keep the busy beasts inside you active.
- Be kind to strangers and other people, including your own family and friends. Sometimes, just realizing that not everything is about you gives you a perspective into things. A global pandemic didn't happen to keep you from enjoying your honeymoon in the Maldives. Instead of doing a Karen or Ken,

volunteer at a charitable agency delivering food and groceries to vulnerable, elderly people. That ought to knock some sense into you that you have so much more to live for than wallowing in your frustration and several gallons of sweet tea.

- Unplug from all your gadgets. Get off the grid and enjoy a whole weekend of no doomscrolling, trolling, fake news, and senseless repeats of dumb dance moves. Give yourself a chance to detox from hours upon hours of screentime and human-to-human toxicity. Refocus your attention to the natural colors around you, the ebb and flow of rural or urban life, the buzz of honeybees. Seek tranquillity when and where you can.

This is by no means an exhaustive list, but it's a start. There's enough inspiration here to get your own mind churning out ideas, leaving no time for you to consider three large burritos from the food truck at the end of your street. There are so many activities out there to engage in. Whatever you decide on that works for you, just make sure that you're managing your emotions the right way. It bears repeating here that acting out your stress by bullying others isn't one of them. Neither is playing the game of mythical monkeys (see nothing, hear nothing, say nothing aka denial) nor ghosting the world as you retreat into your own private hideaway. You conceal your problematic emotions and they'll just fester away behind the curtain.

For sure, your real needs don't want you to embark on a journey of self-harm either. Bingeing on food is one example. The fact that it makes you feel guilty and ashamed is proof enough that it's not and will never be the solution to your needs. The same goes for substance abuse. Whether it's alcohol, meth, or opiates, substances are not fairy dust to set you free; they're a tether to enslave you for a long time unless you get help.

Giving in to your real needs is not like throwing yourself into a mosh pit and trusting that someone or something is going to break your fall when you jump off the stage. Your best bet is to be mindful about every step you take as you address your needs. Before you give in to the contents of your pantry, never forget that "pause" is a legitimate and acceptable action to your ricocheting emotions. Press pause and drop everything that you're doing and say hi to them. Know them. Own them.

After acknowledging your emotions, give yourself time to think about them. Try to understand what they are and what you can do to deal with them. If it feels like you can't take care of them on your own, reach out to somebody who can assist you. You may need professional help outrightly or just basic quality time from your family and close friends. Don't second-guess the latter and talk yourself out of asking them for help because you think they'll disdain you. Allow them to respond on their own. Just be sure to let them know your situation because they can't read your mind or discern your private affairs. If they're your people, of course, they'll open their arms wide and be there for you. Then you'll know that you've surrounded yourself with the best support circle. Emotional eating won't stand a chance against such a formidable support team and resources.

A long time ago, I had a friend who was a superathlete. She excelled in a variety of team and individual sports like volleyball and table tennis. She was fit and heading for an adult life full of adventures, climbing rocks, hiking mountains, and cycling through forest trails. One day, she injured her back and had to undergo a long period of rehabilitation. During her time of helplessness, she also started a relationship with someone who showed her love and affection by cooking all her favorite foods, among other things. Her partner was such a huge help for her, walking up the stairs, changing her clothes, and driving her around everywhere that she humored him by eating all the food he cooked for her. She was often stuffed to the point of vomiting, but she held it all in because he was a good guy and needed him around to provide her mobility.

Eventually, they did break up, but my friend's inclination to eat never stopped until she ballooned to a point that she could no longer play the sports she loved without feeling sluggish and inept. Finally, when a life-threatening condition reared up its ugly head to curtail her freedom further, she decided to put a stop to her destructive eating behavior. With the help of a therapist, a cheering squad of loved ones, and multiple alternative activities, she slowly reduced her weight closer and closer to where it could be safe for her to get physically active again. She realized that she had transmogrified food and eating into entities of connection, certainty, and significance in her mind so much that she had become a slave to them. She felt loved and a reason to love through food. She felt so much pleasure while eating because she felt her every "need" met. She felt like the center of the world when someone doted on her hand and foot by feeding her.

Over time, my friend has learned to be better at keeping in touch with other people. Instead of being completely co-dependent (another issue for another day and book) and fixated on a single person, she allowed her social circle to be more inclusive and diverse. She hangs out with a different group of people

CONQUER EMOTIONAL EATING | 131

who share her passion for camping, but she never misses family gatherings. She has broadened her pastime to include gardening, so she could still be outdoors without straining her still-recovering body. When she's especially feeling antsy about not being able to climb mountains—yet—she takes a spade, trowel, rake, and seed packets, putting some good distance between the kitchen and herself. Before sleeping, she writes in her journal, detailing things she's happy about that day. She no longer identifies herself with what she eats. Her life has become so much more interesting and multidimensional than that.

To date, she still hasn't reached her healthy target weight, but my friend is getting there. She still enjoys her food a lot, but she no longer treats it like a life raft. It's her nourishment, yes, but it has no connection to her emotions. She keeps both of them in separate cubicles and hopes they never meet again for the rest of her lifetime.

If you're currently struggling with an urge to eat your emotions, look over the list of suggested alternatives and try one or two of them on yourself. Write down the details of how you got them started and what your gut reaction was to each of them. Try to flip through your earlier journal entries and see if your chosen alternatives address any of the needs you noted in the past.

Every time you attempt a substitute to food for your fulfillment of needs, note it down and compare it to previous alternates. Celebrate little steps that take you away from emotional eating and into a freedom to eat healthily and happily.

7

OBSERVE AND OBEY YOUR TRUE HUNGER

Food is more than just an incredible source of nourishment for any human being. It also brings a lot of pleasure, comfort, and other good feels into our bodies, minds, and spirits that there's no way you can completely do away with it in your life.

When I started this book on overcoming emotional eating, the end was never to eliminate food from your life or even to restrict you to yet another diet but to put food in its proper place and to offer you more options for dealing with your emotions besides eating. You're still absolutely free to enjoy all your meals, snacks, and treats. That's not the issue. The questions you need to answer at this point are these: Can you relish eating without going overboard and becoming an emotional eater again? Are you able to treat food as nourishment without eventually making it into an emotional crutch? What steps can you take, so you don't fall into the old pattern ever again?

These questions aren't easily answered, considering that you can never tell what each day may bring. It's been recorded that people who follow the Alcoholics Anonymous program sometimes fall off the wagon even after two decades of sobriety. That's the nature of their disease and how life happens. If emotional eating has been your default mode for much of your existence, then you may expect things to be touch-and-go in the beginning until you get the hang of it. It may take a while for you to change over completely, so set your expectations at the right level to avoid frustration and despair at yourself. The only guarantee you have is what you can control in front of you at this very moment, today.

In an earlier section of the book, I had mentioned about mindful eating and this is the tool you currently have available to you in your shed. You probably didn't even know it existed or was already within your reach. Mindful eating is your ability to appreciate all the benefits eating brings to your body and tapping all of them to keep you well-nourished, healthy, and strong. It's the practice of carefully selecting and savoring food that satisfies your senses and bodily needs. Mindful eating is also a kind of discipline as you learn to listen to your body and be appropriately responsive to the cues it gives you, regarding hunger and fullness.

Mindful eating is not a new thing. If anything, it's simply a return to how our human ancestors used to enjoy their food—as many people, including me, imagined them doing it: without any distraction, without multitasking, and for the primary reason of nourishing their bodies and feeding their physical hunger. At a time when they were hunting and gathering organically —learning which were edible and which brought illness or death on the spot, without any referential point other than their real-time experience—mindful eating had to be their operating system because they were just then getting to know the world and how things worked in it.

And so, we fast-forward to the present. You may often miss the point of eating these days because it's merely another item in your to-do list, squeezed between yoga class and picking up the kids from soccer practice. That's the trap of mindless eating. When you chow down on a bagel while driving or riding the train to your workplace, when you poke your fork into a Chinese oyster pail at your desk while filling out cells on an Excel spreadsheet, or when you take giant gulps of Slurpee while in the middle of a hot chase in Grand

Theft Auto, your attention is everywhere but on your food. Because you're not keeping track of how your body responds to it, you miss so many indicators of when you've had enough or when you still need more or whether you're eating the right kind of food to begin with. All this has got to change if you want to put emotional eating squarely in your rear-view mirror.

Thankfully, the steps for putting emotional eating behind you are not difficult to follow. You just need to commit yourself to them and be patient with yourself when you make mistakes or fall short of your own expectations. At various times in the book's earlier chapters, I had actually already given examples to you about what mindful eating is all about and what it looks like. In this chapter, I'll recap them and elaborate further on a few points.

Mindful eating is about being in the present and being fully in control of your eating experience. You do not switch your body over to autopilot. It's manual all the way, okay? You are conscious of how you're poised over your food, what meal is in front of you, how things are arranged on the table. Everything before you is there by your own deliberate design. Nothing is random. You have sparkling water by choice, not because you "settled" for whatever you can find in the fridge. It's what you really want to have for that homemade dinner.

Even the contents of your fridge and pantry are ingredients and other foodstuff that you want for your nourishment, not because they were on sale at the supermarket.

Regardless of how you transport food from your plate to your mouth—spoon, fork, knife, chopsticks, hand—mindful eating unfolds at a calculated, slow pace. If it were music, it would be adagio, not allegro, vivace, presto, or faster. You are not under threat of having your stockpile of food stolen by a pack of ravenous scavenger wolves. You have no business thoughtlessly stuffing your face like a resource-guarding rescue dog. It's unfortunate that you can't simply throw a ball onto your plate to reduce your eating speed the way experienced dog owners do for their pets, but that's exactly what you need to do—not the ball thing but the slowing down thing.

Mindful eating encourages you to cut a morsel slowly and bring it to your mouth when the latter is completely empty—its previous contents fully swallowed and washed down by some form of liquid. It's not just bad etiquette to put a spoonful in when you're still chewing, but it's also a choking accident waiting to happen. There is no overlapping of actions in mindful eating. One thing follows after the other in a linear fashion. The only layering you have will be that of the fundamental but complex flavors of your food—its acid, fat, heat, and salt, according to a New York Times bestselling book.

Mindful eating means that you focus on the tastes of your food. You will never be able to appreciate them when you're chewing faster than an F1 McLaren-Honda on an Italian racecourse. Eating needs to be a stand-alone activity in your schedule, so you never miss out on the best things about food. If you happen to be your own home chef, all the more reason to carve out time and space for cooking and meals. You're not going to be that cook who slaps anything and everything together, hoping for an edible miracle to come out of your efforts. You want to be that thoughtful one who blends ingredients together in a coherent, healthy composition. When other people say that they're way too busy to cook and eat slowly, I think to myself, "Maybe you're not actually busy. You just need to pause and assess the hierarchy of your to-dos more carefully."

At some point, you need to realize that eating and other allied activities (such as cooking) shouldn't be negotiable. They mustn't be the ones always to suffer being pushed around or canceled altogether in your schedule. In a measurable way, your life depends on them. Humans can supposedly survive only up to a week with no food and no water. Eating (and drinking are) is essential to your survival, so don't treat it like an afterthought, aside, or mere time-killer.

When you're eating, don't let your mind wander off, if you can help it. Worrying about pending work won't make it go away. You just need to deal with it after dining. I know a few families that ban all electronic gadgets from their dining table during meals. If that's what it takes for you to be in the moment of eating, then let it be so. Switch off the TV. Play some soft, light music or not at all. Set up your dining area so that eating together with other people or by yourself becomes a pleasant experience, one that is conducive for slowing down, one that you look forward to. Of course, the ideal situation is to eat together with family and friends. Being alone can sometimes take away your sense of accountability, so you may end up overdoing the portions on your plate.

When eating mindfully, you can prepare yourself by taking slow, deep breaths before digging in. You are setting the stage for you being in full control of your body. It's always best to sit down while eating. It's a restful position and that's how you should be enjoying your food—while you're at rest.

To control the pace of your eating, set your utensils down and concentrate on chewing. Sources vary on the number of times you should chew, but I personally recommend 20 to 30 chews before swallowing. The act of chewing isn't just so you could enjoy the variety of flavors in your food; it's also to trigger the process of digestion right in your mouth. Your saliva contains vital enzymes that help you digest food. When you barely chew, your saliva has no chance of mixing in with the food to add in the said enzymes. Chewing also allows the food to lose its original texture, so that it becomes much smoother and easier to transport throughout your digestive system. Yet another benefit of chewing is eliminating or lowering the potential for choking. When you chew, you make food pieces small enough to pass through the tight spaces of your esophagus, intestines, etc., without causing a traffic jam. With this in mind, it's also advisable to have bite-sized pieces on your plate.

Don't just eat for your sense of taste; eat to stimulate all the rest of your senses. This is a secret that top chefs the world over have known all this time. Food is meant to excite your eyes, nose, ears, and touch, too. The sound of sizzling on a hot cast-iron platter is often enough to make true-blue carnivores drool before they even see, smell, or taste the black peppercorn steak approaching from behind them. The feeling of warm sweat dripping down the side of your face is part of the experience when eating Szechuan cuisine and its predominantly peppery dishes. Notice how much more satiated you are when you allow yourself to absorb these food nuances. You stay full longer and the memory is something that you can keep coming back to days or even years after the experience.

Mindful eating teaches you not to castigate yourself for your responses to food. There's no judgment when you love ice cream, hate ratatouille, or have no opinion about matcha tea, regardless of what your woke hipster friends say about it. As a Latin maxim states, *"De gustibus non est disputandum."* You don't fight over differing tastes, even with yourself and certainly not with other people. "Healthy food" doesn't look the same for every person, so don't feel bad that you simply can't stand Greek salad but appreciate an Ethiopian mixed platter, with both veggie and meat dishes arranged on a single, large piece of teff injera.

Your enjoyment of food ultimately makes its way to your metaphorical heart, where your emotions reside, but this is by no means a sign that food feeds your emotions. It simply means that you have eaten so well and so happily that the positive effect goes deep down into your innermost being. Your emotions become the recipient of the good feels from food. They are not the cause for you to eat food. And because mindful eating can result in such an upbeat state of being, you eventually find yourself making choices that truly benefit you.

You don't need to put yourself on a diet anymore. You naturally seek food and fall into eating habits that are pro-you, that lead you to grow as a person in more than just your physical aspect.

Mindful eating gives you full control of the wheel. As you listen to your body, you become much more aware of what is good and not good for it, and you respond accordingly. You make choices based on good, solid information provided by your body. You don't have other people telling you what to eat and what not to eat. Your body knows. If you allow your body to relish the food you give it, it will communicate to you loudly and clearly when its full or when it needs more. It will tell you that you're feeding it too much processed sugar and not enough fruits and vegetables.

Mindful eating makes you aware that your eating habits and food connect you to the environment at large. You choose to eat a Ugandan dark chocolate bar not only because it's absolutely heavenly but because it is processed by hand, left a small carbon footprint, and is a fairtrade product. You don't drink a certain coffee brand because they've been known to use child laborers for the harvest of their beans. Those are the kinds of connections that matter and which mindful eating brings to the table.

What remains now is this question: how do you know when you're truly physically hungry? Emotional hunger often masquerades as physical hunger, so this can be a real worry for you. You don't want to be conned into eating before it's time, but you also don't want to wait too long before eating because it can lead to overeating, stomach cramps, and other ill effects.

If you're physically hungry, the sensation will build up and come to you over time, maybe several hours after your last food intake. Be suspicious of hunger that comes suddenly out of nowhere. Physical hunger will manifest to you in tangible ways. A growling stomach is one of them, caused by the contraction of your digestive organs, such as the stomach and intestines. If your stomach feels empty, that's another sign that it's time for your body to eat.

Hangry isn't just a fancy portmanteau for being angry because you're hungry. It's a genuine phenomenon because you can indeed become irritable if your physical hunger isn't immediately addressed. You may also find yourself with a headache, which instantly disappears as soon as you start eating. It's important not to delay the satiation of your physical hunger because you don't want to suffer from fatigue and a mental concentration deficit.

While I do encourage a quick response to physical hunger, that doesn't mean that you're at its beck and call, ergo, a slave to it. You should still be able to exercise a degree of control over physical hunger. A drink of cold water can certainly do the trick. Take one glass of it before every meal. Another practical way of controlling your physical hunger is to use smaller plates. Many people embark on a see-food diet, so they tend to fill up their plates to overflowing for as long as there's food in front of them and there's an empty space on their plate. A smaller one ensures that people get sober portions for themselves. Even a simple thing as cutting up your food gives the illusion of "more" on your plate. On that note, you should also serve and eat finger foods (including chips, crackers, and nuts) from bowls or saucers, so you can see the amounts you're shoving into your mouth. When taken from their original (opaque) packaging, you can never tell just how much you're already ingesting before it's too late and the bag is empty.

Sometimes, you may not always be in a position to satisfy physical hunger instantaneously because you're not in the right time and place. Remember, you also want to exercise mindful eating when you can finally sit down to eat, so a quickie doesn't work. You must be able to situate yourself in such a way that you're not going to be rushed or reckless with your food choice.

By the same measure that I encourage you to understand your emotional hunger, I encourage you to do the
same when it comes to physical hunger. According to
the American Diabetes Association, there are at least 10
steps that separate sheer hunger from overeating. Here
is their hunger-satiety scale:

Full	10 =	Stuffed to the point of feeling sick
	9 =	Very uncomfortably full, need to loosen your belt
	8 =	Uncomfortably full, feel stuffed
	7 =	Very full, feel as if you have overeaten
	6 =	Comfortably full, satisfied
Neutral	5 =	Comfortable, neither hungry nor full
	4 =	Beginning signs and symptoms of hunger
	3 =	Hungry with several hunger symptoms, ready to eat
	2 =	Very hungry, unable to concentrate
Hungry	1 =	Starving, dizzy, irritable

Based on the information above, you don't really want
to go below level three of the scale. As soon as
multiple hunger symptoms start manifesting themselves, you must create time and space for your
mindful eating. It's rather unfortunate that hangry has
become such a popular term because it means that
many people deprive themselves of food past the
acceptable point. You must strive to eliminate that
word from your vocabulary by paying attention to
your body and not pushing the limits of its endurance.
It's especially important that you don't wait too long

to eat when you have a condition that requires you to do so at the right time. You also don't want to go to the extreme and overfeed yourself. Hitting levels eight, nine, or 10 sounds like a lot of trouble to deal with. Again, they will have a negative effect on your body and that's not what food and eating are supposed to generate.

Your sweet spot in the scale is somewhere in the middle, where you can fully enjoy your food without guilt, worry, or fear. You eat it at the right time, in the right place, at the right amount, and at the right pace. You eat because your body told you so, not because your emotions were crushing you into submission. It's a beautiful thing to know that you are the master of your eating, isn't it? When you can see it from this perspective, conquering emotional eating indeed becomes feasible.

Mindful eating isn't about losing weight or dieting, but it can certainly benefit you in that regard, if that's something you desperately need to do. Just ask Melanie, for instance. For the longest time, Melanie never considered herself in dire straits when it came to her weight. She was in full body-positive mode, so she was not interested in anyone telling her that she was overweight. But then she started having the worst series of acid reflux in her personal history. When consulted, her physician told her that she was not in a healthy weight and needed to trim her frame down.

At first, Melanie was resistant to the idea, but as her acid reflux worsened, she decided to try something. She wasn't interested in diets, so a friend told her to practice mindful eating instead. She still ate the same types of food, but as she became more conscious of what and how she ate, she saw many ways by which she could rein in her eating. She put only enough on her plate. She chewed her food more thoroughly. She kept her phone in her pocket. She deliberated over her food and didn't settle for "whatever is there".

As Melanie continued changing little things about her eating habits, she started noticing the difference. She no longer had to pop open the button of her jeans after a full meal. Her food tasted leagues better when she sat still and enjoyed it. Her stomach stopped feeling bloated every time she ate. There were several other welcome changes, but the one she cherished the most was the elimination of her acid reflux. Her diet still included a lot of dairy and meats, but they were now in small portions, proportional to her physical hunger and nothing else. This most certainly can be your story, too. I'm not saying that you need to lose weight, okay? But Melanie's story can inspire anybody who wishes to make healthy changes for the good of their bodies.

Mindful eating does that and more. It helps you enjoy food to the fullest—with pun intended.

As I close this chapter, I'd like you to try these exercises whenever you find yourself eating carelessly. They are meant to take your attention back to the act of eating and be present in it once again:

- Retreat to a dark corner, sit down, close your eyes, and bite down on your food. Or just simply shut your eyes and eat. Deprive yourself of visual delights, so your mind can reset and focus only on your eating. This way, you can hear better when you're already full. You can count the number of times you chew. You're in the moment and nothing else is going to take you away from it, so enjoy.
- Eat with your non-dominant hand. If you're righthanded, be a leftie at mealtimes. And vice versa. This prevents you from finishing your food before your body says enough; you automatically slow down as you struggle to hold your utensils. Fumbling with your chopsticks is good. It keeps you grounded in the eating process.
- Disrupt the queue of incoming flavors. If you're enjoying the bowl of potato chips way too much, switch over to a different food, so you

don't lose yourself in the yummy flavors that keep coming at you on cue. Throw in wasabi-flavored nuts in there. Take a moment to let that wasabi creep up your nose like a ninja before going back to your chips. Hopefully, the disruption actually causes you to stop eating chips, so your mindless eating also ceases. Absolutely nothing wrong, of course, with what you're eating, but you now have to learn the how of eating to complete your mastery over food.

8

PRACTICAL WAYS TO SUPPORT HEALTHY EATING

Writing this book has been a wonderful adventure for me because I had you in mind. If it is to be worth all the long hours in front of my laptop and more long hours in practicing what I preach, it has to find real-time application in your daily life. This is the hope I have as I write this last chapter.

By now, you've reached the end of the LET GO method. To recap, the acronym stands for the following:

- Lead your thoughts.
- Evade your triggers.
- Tune in to your emotions.
- Give in to your real needs.
- Observe and obey your true hunger.

All these statements are, of course, in relation to the main objective of this book: to give you the principles and tools you need to overcome emotional eating. While it may all seem overwhelming right now, you just need to take a small step a day at a time to reach your goal. It's very important to have a goal, so you know the direction for applying all your time, energy, and other resources. Emotional eating is not your average challenge. It will take your whole being to counter its negative effects in your life. You need to be deliberate and prepared when you deal with it, hence, the goal setting. You will not be Don Quixote tilting at the windmill. You will be Frodo heading for Mordor.

When it comes to goals, don't go crazy and plan for a hundred. You're better off with just three that are well within your powers to accomplish than an ambitious hundred that are more for preening than actual execution. Make them SMART goals—specific, measurable, achievable, realistic, and time-bound. Once your few goals are set, create action steps to make them attainable. You don't just become a Dragon Warrior after a good-night's sleep. Po the Panda needed to undergo a long, grueling kung-fu training regimen under Master Shifu before he could become his destiny as a legendary hero.

When it comes to goals for changing your behavior, ground them as close to reality as possible. You're not wishing upon a star here or having a fairy dream. You want to make something happen. You want to change. For real. You can't get more authentic than letting your goal reflect what you truly want for yourself. It's also helpful if your goal connects with your many interests. See how you can incorporate your love for the outdoors in it. Or your desire for do-gooding. You're more likely to reach your goal when you're vested in it. It's a perfect setup for success.

A behavioral-change goal requires a commitment to discipline, a huge hurdle for many. Discipline requires you to practice a strict adherence to a particular code of conduct, something that you may not be willing to subject yourself to. If you reach the point where you must sit down with your emotions to get to know them, you can't abscond. You either do it and do it well or just forget about conquering emotional eating altogether. That's not negotiable. There are other things along the way that you can compromise on, but you must also be willing to recognize the ones that you can't. Know the difference.

When it comes to setting yourself up for success, you need to look beyond yourself and evaluate your environment. Is everything nice and kosher for mindful eating or do you need to level up your game? Take a moment to read up on good nutrition. If this is your first time to cook beyond frying and boiling, then go ahead and buy a recipe book on healthy dishes. It's not about going vegetarian or vegan either. It's about using nutritious ingredients you'll love to eat. There's a whole world of delicious food out there, which aren't laden with just butter and 10 kinds of cheese.

If it comes down to this, be willing to overhaul the contents of your pantry, fridge, and freezer. And anywhere else where you store food—your car's glove compartment or the bottom drawer of your office desk. Stock up on a variety of cereals and grains. Corn flakes aren't the only breakfast cereals in the world. Discover muesli and even the humble oats. Overnight oats are not new, but there are people out there who still haven't heard about it, possibly including you. You don't need to be a professional nutritionist to know what to eat and what not to eat. Just turn the package over and read the labels. Watch out for too much sugar, artificial flavoring, additives, etc.

A basic knowledge of health from your home economics class should tell you that your body needs fiber from fruits and vegetables, that you can get "good fat" from avocado, that roasting can make meat just as tasty as frying, but with less grease. In other words, you can't claim ignorance when it comes to collecting truthful and reliable information. Know as much as possible about a healthy lifestyle from trustworthy sources. Libraries, government websites, universities, and established media outlets are good places to start your research.

A lifestyle change can be as simple as taking away every filled candy dish readily available around your house. Don't make it easy for you to access food that can lead to mindless eating. Put all your chocolates on the top shelf of your pantry. Don't buy supersized bags of this or that snack. If you must because they're cheaper, at least divide them into smaller containers at home. Minimize your purchase of processed foods. Don't go grocery shopping when you're a volcano of emotions. It's going to lead you to the valley of the shadow of unhealthy foods and that'll just unleash new demons from the town of guilt and shame. When your emotions are in turmoil, remember to press pause.

Also, don't make it a habit to eat out regularly. Nothing wrong in eating out, but you want to master your emotional eating. It's just one way of minimizing your exposure to triggers. It's very easy to forget and let your guard down when the buffet tables are just a few feet away from you at an all-you-can-eat restaurant. Keep things moderate, even when you have the disposable income for it.

A very effective way of slamming the door on the face of emotional eating is to plan and prepare your meals. If you know you're heading out into the wilderness, you get ready in advance. That's pretty much Scouting 101. You bring enough water, sun protection, trail mixes, etc. way before you even climb into a vehicle and drive off. Meal planning and preparation is you getting ready for your own kind of "wilderness trek". Say, if you know that the coming work week is going to be toxic because of a project deadline, then schedule a couple of hours on the Sunday before to cook a batch of dishes to cover you from Monday to the next weekend. Don't allow yourself to settle for fast food or takeaway because that's just encouraging mindless munching. You'll be too tired and too stressed even to notice it.

Before you can get into a meal plan for a toxic week ahead, it pays to have the right ingredients already within arm's reach. A few paragraphs earlier, I had hinted at the possibility of revamping the contents of your pantry, fridge, and freezer. If you had been scratching your head all this time as to how that's supposed to look like, this is where your guesswork ends. You don't even have to trawl Trader Joe's for fancy-shmancy foodstuff.

Let's start with your condiments. Consider stocking up on the following items:

- Dijon mustard as base for salad dressings
- Maple syrup as sweetener for dishes and drinks and as topping for breakfast food (go for the pure one, not the ones laden with corn syrup and other additives)
- Soy sauce for the umami in anything you can think of (aim for the low-sodium variety)
- Tahini as a unique flavor addition to soups, salad dressings, pastries, and meats

Besides your usual meats, fish, and seafood for protein sources, have the subsequent ingredients on hand:

- Eggs for quick-cook solutions
- Nuts and nut butters for snacks, sandwiches, and dishes
- Tofu as meat substitute or protein supplement in dishes and drinks

These are dairy products your pantry shouldn't be without:

- Cheese—no explanation needed, I'm sure
- Dairy milk or plant-based alternatives (like almond, soy, or oats)—again, no explanation needed
- Greek yogurt as a healthier substitute for sour cream, best in plain version (you can also use plant-based ones)

The following fresh produce pack a punch in terms of vitamins and minerals and can blend in with whatever meal you have planned for the day:

- Apples
- Avocados
- Bananas
- Basil, cilantro, and other fresh herbs
- Beans and peas
- Berries of all kinds
- Canned fruits and vegetables (in water or their own juice)
- Carrots
- Celery
- Cruciferous vegetables (bok choy, broccoli, cauliflower, etc.)

- Cucumbers
- Kale, lettuce, and other leafy greens
- Lemons and limes
- Oranges
- Peppers
- Potatoes
- Raisins
- Squash
- Tomatoes

Grains and cereals should also be present in your pantry because they have fiber, minerals, and more in them, necessary for digestion and other bodily functions. The list below is by no means exhaustive, but it's a start:

- Brown rice
- Chickpeas
- Popcorn
- Quinoa
- Tortillas
- Whole-grain breads and crackers

You don't have to stock up on all of these foodstuffs, of course, but if you can have even just a fraction of them ready for your meal planning, then you can already take those small steps toward healthier eating.

Now we move on to meal planning. Take time to list down your favorite meals. If you have a family, include each individual's as well. You can combine dishes or highlight a favorite for the day. You can spread the favorite meals across the week. After all, you have three meals to plan for daily—plenty of opportunities to accommodate everyone. Have a bit of adventure and try something new from reading recipe books or sites. A key criterion is to create variety to your meals. Not everything has to be soup. Not everything has to be grilled. You don't always have to have meat or go full vegetarian. Everybody has their respective dietary requirements, so always strive to find the middle ground. If you're planning for just yourself, then you only have your own needs to take care of. Your grocery list will be based on the meals you have planned. In the long run, meal planning gives you more than just a pathway to healthy eating; it also helps you save money. You minimize random purchases and possibly pay wholesale prices for ingredients used in several dishes.

Well-planned meals are always well-balanced in terms of nutrition and simplicity. You're not doing an Iron Chef episode, competing against the greatest chefs in the world. Cook dishes that you'll actually consume. Don't be like this guy who cooked an elaborate coq au vin dish only to throw away almost half of it. No one else in his family liked it and he had ambitiously doubled the measurements of ingredients. Make just enough food to keep wastage low.

With low food wastage in mind, know that some ingredients can't survive meal preparation very well. Avoid fruits and veggies like avocado and lettuce, for instance, because they're too soft and don't keep long once cut and stored. If you must have them, just allow yourself a few minutes to prep them on the day that you need them. Don't linger. The point of meal prep is to save on time.

Not all your meals have to be cooked, especially if that toxic work week coming up is going to steal away all your downtime. It's sensible to plan for quick-prep foods like sandwiches or wraps. You still get the same amount of nutrients and calories from them that you would otherwise get from cooked dishes—if you plan well. Once your meal plan is in place, stick to the schedule. Don't forget to account for any restaurant meals for someone's special day. You obviously can't say no to all dine-out engagements, just be sure to make the appropriate adjustments for that day in terms of how much you eat and what time to eat.

Beyond the meal plan itself, maximize your hours by doing the planning, grocery shopping, and cooking/prepping all on the same day. It saves time and effort for you, especially if you also organize your shopping in such a way that you go aisle by targeted aisle, not zigzag through the entire supermarket. Having all that done together also helps you be mindful about food and eating. No distractions from other parts of your life to pull you in 10 different directions.

By the same way that you should shop methodically, you should also do the same with your meal preparations, including the cooking part. If five meals call for chopped onions, do all of it in one go rather than chopping one per meal. If certain dishes require longer cooking times, do them first before you tackle the no-cook ones. The stewing, baking, and whatever can happen in the background while you go about storing ingredients for assembling later into sandwiches, wraps, etc.

Meal planning and prepping can be a game changer in your efforts at healthy living. Not only can you exercise portion control, but you can also manage your kitchen/food waste better and save more moolah for that dream vacation to the Caribbean. It's not a vanity thing. You actually can't get more pragmatic than this when it comes to food and eating.

In case you're floundering about, not knowing where to begin, here's a one-week sample meal plan for you to try:

Monday

▷ Breakfast

- 1 tangerine
- 2 large eggs (boiled, poached, or fried)
- 1 slice whole-grain toast

▷ Morning Snack

- 1 banana
- 1 cup Greek yogurt with 1 tablespoon maple syrup

▷ Lunch

- 4 ounces grilled chicken breast (skinless and boneless)
- 2 cups mixed greens salad, topped with tomatoes, avocado, balsamic vinaigrette

▷ Afternoon Snack

- 1 medium carrot
- 3 tablespoons hummus

▷ Dinner

- 1 cup broccoli (cooked to your taste)
- 1/2 cup cooked brown rice (although white won't be a deal breaker)
- 4 ounces white-meat fish fillet

Tuesday

▷ Breakfast

- 1 orange
- 2 tablespoons nut butter
- 1 whole-wheat muffin

▷ Morning Snack

- 1/2 cup berries
- 1 cup Greek yogurt

▷ Lunch

- Turkey sandwich (4 ounces turkey breast, 1 large tomato slice, lettuce leaves, avocado, 2 teaspoons mustard, 2 slices whole-wheat bread)

▷ Afternoon Snack

- 1 cup grapes

▷ Dinner

- 3 ounces steak (your choice of part)
- 1 small roasted sweet potato
- 1/2 cup spinach (cooked to your taste)
- 1/2 cup green beans (cooked to your taste)

Wednesday

▷ Breakfast

- overnight oats (1 mashed banana, 2 tablespoons cashew nuts, 1 tablespoon raisins, 1/2 cup oats, 1 cup milk, 1/3 cup Greek yogurt)

▷ Morning Snack

- 1 fresh pear
- 22 almonds

▷ Lunch

- 1 fried egg
- 1 slice whole-wheat bread

- 1/2 cup mashed avocado
- 1 medium apple

▷ Afternoon Snack

- 3 tablespoons hummus
- 1 cup carrots
- 1 cup tomatoes

▷ Dinner

- 1 whole-wheat muffin
- 4 ounces turkey burger patty
- 1 tomato slice, 2 lettuce leaves, 1 onion slice
- 2 tablespoons ketchup

Thursday

▷ Breakfast

- 2 slices whole-wheat bread
- 2 tablespoons nut butter
- 1 banana

▷ Morning Snack

- 1 cup grapes
- 14 walnuts

▷ Lunch

- 1 tuna wrap (1 wheat-flour tortilla, 1/2 can tuna in water but drained, 1 tablespoon mayo, lettuce, tomato)

▷ Afternoon Snack

- 1 cup cottage cheese
- 1/2 cup berries

▷ Dinner

- 1 cup whole-wheat pasta
- 1 cup tomato sauce
- 1 cup mixed greens salad, topped with tomatoes and balsamic vinaigrette

Friday

▷ Breakfast

- 1 cup Greek yogurt
- ¾ cup blueberries
- 2 tablespoons almonds

▷ Morning Snack

- 1/2 cup carrots
- 1/2 cup cauliflower
- 2 tablespoons ranch dip

▷ Lunch

- 1 veggie burger patty
- 1 whole-grain bun
- 1 slice cheddar cheese
- 1 apple

▷ Afternoon Snack

- 1 banana
- 2 tablespoons nut butter

▷ Dinner

- 4 ounces white-meat fish fillet
- 1 cup steamed beans
- 1/2 cup cooked brown rice (again, white won't be a deal breaker)
- 1 cup mixed greens salad, topped with tomatoes and balsamic vinaigrette

Saturday

▷ Breakfast

- 1 cup Greek yogurt
- 1 banana
- 1 hard-boiled egg

▷ Morning Snack

- 10 whole-wheat pretzel bites
- 3 tablespoons hummus

▷ Lunch

- 1 tortilla wrap (1 piece whole-wheat tortilla, 4 ounces turkey, 1 slice cheddar cheese, 1 cup mixed greens, 1 tablespoon honey mustard)

▷ Afternoon Snack

- 11 almonds
- 1 fresh peach

▷ Dinner

- 4 ounces pork loin
- 1 small baked potato

- 5 asparagus stalks
- 1 cup mixed greens salad, topped with tomatoes and balsamic vinaigrette

Sunday

▷ Breakfast

- 1 cup cooked oats
- 1/2 cup berries
- 1/2 cup milk
- 2 tablespoons nut butter

▷ Morning Snack

- 1 cup Greek yogurt
- 1 apple

▷ Lunch

- 4 ounces baked chicken breast
- 2 cups mixed greens salad, topped with tomatoes, onions, balsamic vinaigrette
- 1 baked sweet potato

▷ Afternoon Snack

- 1 cup raw broccoli

- 1 cup carrots
- 3 tablespoons hummus

▷ Dinner

- 4 ounces salmon fillet (grilled, baked, or to your taste)
- 1/2 cup cooked brown rice
- 5 asparagus stalks

The meal plan presented here is just a basic framework. You can improvise as you go. For instance, since I don't specify which berries to use, you have the field open to strawberries, blueberries, blackberries, and the like. For the white-meat fish, you have cod, halibut, flounder, and more. You can try hummus with pine nuts or garlic. Bottom line, the meal plan is for you, so you make it fit your tastes, with the view of giving yourself the healthiest meals that bring pleasure, too.

An authentic transformation in your life is not a pipe dream. For as long as you're committed to the journey, the little tweaks you make here and there can add up to a compelling and welcome story of change. You won't even be alone to celebrate it. Many people who have cheered you on all this time will be there and it'll be one heck of a celebration for everybody.

Claire was a slim, tiny lady who was well-loved by all because she was an achiever in many fields of her adult life. She was a responsible and trusted employee in a corporation, where she rose up the ranks fairly quickly because of her impeccable work ethic. She was an active community member and could be counted on to volunteer for many initiatives that benefited the most vulnerable people in her area. She was everybody's favorite aunt when family gathered together because she always remembered their special days and gifted them with something thoughtful.

While she projects an aura of confidence to the people around her, in private, Claire was an emotional wreck. She was a certified introvert, but the world had seemingly conspired to put her in the forefront of many things. She was never comfortable speaking in front of a group of people. She was deathly scared of idle chitchat in social situations. To counter her fears, doubts, and worries, Claire took to carrying packets of chewing gum anywhere she went and popped one piece out every time she had to emerge from her shell. She easily finished a packet of 10s every couple of hours and replenished her stash round the clock.

Claire eventually developed temporomandibular joint disorder (TMD), which was so severe that it required urgent surgery of her jaws. When her doctor discovered her excessive chewing habit, she was told to see a therapist first to help her deal with how chewing gum ended up becoming her emotional crutch.

Claire was initially irate at the insinuations thrown at her, but she finally owned up to her problem of emotional eating (chewing). She realized that gum had become her main distraction to keep her from focusing on her insecurities, so she had to find a way to deal with them besides falling back on her packet of gum.

With the help of her therapist and a village of people who loved and respected her, Claire learned breathing exercises that calmed her down, discovered music, audiobooks, and podcasts that quieted her fears, and became confident enough to say no occasionally to social invitations that exceeded her capacity for human interaction. She also adopted a dog that kept her company for the moments that she had to be alone and quiet. Claire just needed to do small but consistent changes to her way of life that allowed her finally to let go of her packets of gum and be free to appreciate herself and her life.

Before you move on beyond this book, pick three suggested changes (or variations of them) in this chapter and apply them to your daily life. Create a chart with one column devoted to the three-item list and succeeding columns to correspond to each day of the month chosen (28/29 days for February, 30 days for April, 31 days for December, and so on).

As you progress through the month, place a check mark under each daily column, when you're able to follow through with the change. It's understandable if you miss a few days but do your best to fulfil as many days as possible. At the end of the month, tally up your "on" days and "off" days and evaluate how that change has affected your overall situation. If your changes happen to be related to actual food reduction, calculate how much less calories you've consumed for the month and celebrate the result. Continue on to the next month with a fresh set of three changes and a new chart. Don't slack off on the first three changes though. Carry on with them and enjoy the transformation that results in you.

CONCLUSION

Emotional eating is a real scourge in today's world and many individuals suffer from it—often painfully, alone, and in secret. It is triggered by your emotions that have tricked your mind into believing that food is the answer to your sadness, guilt, pain, and every other negative emotion inside you. When that happens, you run into a whole lot of other problems that compromise your health and well-being.

While there's no fairy godmother who can get rid of emotional eating in your life with just one wave of her magic wand, the LET GO method allows you to gain mastery over your emotions, so you can become a healthier you. The LET GO method has the following key concepts:

- Lead your thoughts.
- Evade your triggers.
- Tune in to your emotions.
- Give in to your real needs.
- Observe and obey your true hunger.

Through the LET GO method, you learn to address your emotions with emotion-based solutions, leaving food to take up its original role as nourishment and pleasure for your physical body. As you practice the LET GO method, you also gain an understanding of mindful eating, which installs the act of eating in its rightful place as something that benefits your physical body, too, in the same way that food does. It does so by situating you firmly in the present as you eat for your bodily sustenance.

As you strengthen your grasp and practice of mindful eating, a positive transformation can happen to your whole being. You are able to control your emotions better, appreciate food and eating as fundamental to your good health and wellbeing, be present in the here and now, and change your circumstances and relationships so that you can carry on mindfully in every aspect of your life for the long term. You just need to LET GO and trust the process.

"What you're supposed to do when you don't like a thing is change it. If you can't change it, change the way you think about it."

— MAYA ANGELOU

If this book has helped you in any way and strikes you as something that can be beneficial to others as well—others who are dealing with their own issues concerning their emotions, actions, and weight—please don't hesitate to leave a review on Amazon. It gives us an opportunity to reach other individuals who may find the insights and advice here significant to their own life journeys.

BIBLIOGRAPHY

Albertson, Ellen. "Be Nicer to Yourself: Using Self-Compassion for Weight Loss Success." Accessed November 12, 2022. https://www.myplenity.com/blog/be-nicer-to-yourself-using-self-compassion

American Diabetes Association. "Get in Touch with Your Appetite." Accessed November 12, 2022. https://diabetes.org/healthy-living/weight-loss/emotions-and-eating/get-touch-your-appetite

Amsellem, Marni. "Understanding and Overcoming Emotional Barriers to Weight Loss." Posted March 23, 2018. https://www.goodtherapy.org/blog/understanding-overcoming-emotional-barriers-to-weight-loss-0323184

Avena, Nicole. "Perfectionism and Self-Criticism." Posted April 27, 2020. https://www.psychologytoday.com/us/blog/food-junkie/202004/perfectionism-and-self-criticism

"Why Do We Eat?" Posted June 17, 2015. https://www.psychologyto day.com/us/blog/food-junkie/201506/why-do-we-eat

Beaumont. "Emotional Eating Conquered through Determination and Support." Posted May 8, 2017. https://www.beaumont.org/health-wellness/news/royal-oak-woman-conquers-emotional-eating-with-determination-and-support .

Beck, Julie. "Our Moods, Our Foods." Posted March 6, 2014. https://www.theatlantic.com/health/archive/2014/03/our-moods-our-foods/284238/

Beckner, Victoria Lemie. "The Key Skill We Rarely Learn: How to Feel Your Feelings." Posted October 12, 2020. https://www.psychology today.com/us/blog/harnessing-principles-change/202010/the-key-skill-we-rarely-learn-how-feel-your-feelings

Bjarnadottir, Adda. "Mindful Eating: A Beginner's Guide." Posted June 19, 2019. https://www.healthline.com/nutrition/mindful-eating guide#intro

Bonvissuto, Danny. "Stock Your Pantry and Refrigerator for Healthy Eating." Accessed November 12, 2022. https://www.webmd.com/diet/healthy-pantry-fridge

Borges, Anna. "9 Emotional Regulation Tips for Anyone Who's Struggling Right Now." Posted May 21, 2020. https://www.self.com/story/emotional-regulation-skills

Bowen, Lisa. "Emotions Are Top Obstacle to Weight Loss, Poll Finds." Posted April 2013. https://www.apa.org/monitor/2013/04/emotions

Brady, Keir. "How to Feel Your Feelings to Improve Your Emotional Well-Being." Accessed November 12, 2022. https://keirbradycounseling.com/feel-your-feelings/

Brissette, Christy. "45 Positive Affirmations to Improve Your Body Image." Accessed November 12, 2022. https://80twentynutrition.com/blog/nutrition-news/positive-affirmations-to-improve-your-body-image/

Brody, Barbara. "How Mindful Eating Helped Me Lose Weight and Love Food." Posted August 29, 2016. https://www.prevention.com/weight-loss/a20472857/how-mindful-eating-helped-me-lose-weight-and-love-food/

Buck, Chad. "Feeding Your Feelings: How Emotions Affect Eating Habits." Accessed November 11, 2022. https://www.vumc.org/health-wellness/news-resource-articles/feeding-your-feelings-how-emotions-affect-eating-habits

Budget Bytes. "Meal Prep 101: A Beginner's Guide to Prepping and Portioning Meals." Accessed November 12, 2022. https://www.budgetbytes.com/meal-prep-101-a-beginners-guide/

Center for Mindful Eating, The. "Introduction to Mindful Eating." Accessed November 12, 2022. https://www.thecenterformindfuleating.org/page-1863947

Centers for Disease Control and Prevention. "Planning Meals." Accessed November 12, 2022. https://www.cdc.gov/healthyweight/healthy_eating/meals.html

Cleveland Clinic. "Mindlessly Snacking (Again)? Try These Simple

Mindful Eating Exercises." Posted October 26, 2020. https://health. clevelandclinic.org/mindlessly-snacking-again-try-these-3-simple-mindful-eating-exercises/

"What Is Emotional Eating?" Posted November 12, 2021. https:// health.clevelandclinic.org/emotional-eating/

"What Is Mindful Eating?" Posted January 31, 2022. https://health. clevelandclinic.org/mindful-eating/

Cuncic, Arlin. "Negative Thoughts: How to Stop Them." Updated October 26, 2021. https://www.verywellmind.com/how-to-change-negative-thinking-3024843

"What Does It Mean to Be 'Triggered'." Updated March 10, 2022. https://www.verywellmind.com/what-does-it-mean-to-be-trig gered-4175432

Evans, Matt. "Real-Life Weight Loss: I Used Food as an Emotional Crutch Until I Discovered Dancing." Posted February 3, 2022. https://www.fitandwell.com/news/rlwl-i-used-food-as-an-emotional-crutch-until-i-discovered-dancing

Feinstein, Kim. "Why Do I Self-Sabotage My Diet?" Accessed November 11, 2022. https://www.redmountainweightloss.com/dr-kim-self-sabotage-controlling-life/

Fit Foodie Life, The. "Emotional Eating: 5 Things You Need to Know." Accessed November 12, 2022. https://www.thefitfoodielife.com/emotional-eating-5-things-to-know/

Flaherty, Rachel. "Weight Loss Became Easier When I Stopped Trying to Be Perfect." Posted February 26, 2019. https://www.irishtimes. com/life-and-style/health-family/fitness/weight-loss-became-easier-when-i-stopped-trying-to-be-perfect-1.3796969

Gilbert, Adam. "A Weight-Loss Expert Explains Why We Sabotage Our Goals (and How to Stop)." Posted October 26, 2017. https://greatist. com/live/weight-loss-tips-how-not-to-self-sabotage#1

Guerdjikova, Anna. "Dangers of Dieting: Why Dieting Can Be Harmful." Posted February 8, 2021. https://lindnercenterofhope.org/blog/why-dieting-can-be-harmful/

Haas, Sara. "17 Healthy Foods to Stock Your Refrigerator." Posted

March 10, 2022. https://www.healthline.com/nutrition/refrigera
tor-food

Harris, Rob. "Self-Discipline in Eating and Exercising." Accessed November 12, 2022. https://www.livestrong.com/article/545644-self-discipline-in-eating-and-exercising/

Harvard Medical School. "8 Steps to Mindful Eating." Posted January 16, 2016. https://www.health.harvard.edu/staying-healthy/8-steps-to-mindful-eating

Healthy Place. "Using Affirmations to Stop Overeating." Updated April 18, 2016. https://motivation.ie/top-tips/positive-affirmations-help-weight-loss/

Help Guide. "Emotional Eating and How to Stop It." Accessed November 11, 2022. https://www.helpguide.org/articles/diets/emotional-eating.htm

Hendel, Hilary Jacobs. "Ignoring Your Emotions Is Bad for Your Health; Here's What to Do About It." Posted February 27, 2018. https://time.com/5163576/ignoring-your-emotions-bad-for-your-health/

Hillary Counseling. "101 Positive Body Affirmations." Accessed November 12, 2022. https://www.hillarycounseling.com/2019/05/02/101-positive-body-affirmations/

Intermountain Healthcare. "Emotional Eating: The Ways We Eat Our Feelings." Accessed November 12, 2022. https://intermountain healthcare.org/ckr-ext/Dcmnt?ncid=529596443

Jurek, Patricia. "Don't Let Negative Self-Talk Sabotage Your Health Goals." Posted August 21, 2017. https://www.henryford.com/blog/2017/08/dont-let-negative-self-talk-sabotage-health-goals

Katz, Terese Weinstein. "Self-Compassion for Weight Loss: 4 Ideas to Help Build It." Posted June 20, 2014. https://www.psychologytoday.com/us/blog/thin-within/201406/self-compassion-weight-loss-4-ideas-help-build-it

Kaushal, Ritu. "Your Feelings Have Messages for You (So Stop Ignoring Them)." Accessed November 12, 2022. https://tinybuddha.com/blog/your-feelings-have-messages-for-you-so-stop-ignoring-them/

Kentucky Counseling Center. "How to Deal with Emotional Triggers." Accessed November 12, 2022. https://kentuckycounselingcenter. com/how-to-deal-with-emotional-triggers/

King, Brian. "Emotional Components of Weight Loss." Posted February 21, 2016. https://www.totalhealthguidance.com/three-emotional-components-of-weight-loss/

Klemz, Joseph. "Achieving Behavior Change through Goal Setting." Accessed November 12, 2022. https://reallifecounseling.us/behav ior-change-goal-setting/

Kravitz, Melissa. "Food Companies Are Making Their Products Addictive and It's Sickening (Literally)." Posted March 26, 2019. https:// www.ecowatch.com/food-companies-making-products-addictive-2632845184.html

Kristenson, Sarah. "65 Affirmations to Help with Your Weight Loss Efforts." Posted November 27, 2021. https://www.happierhuman. com/affirmations-weight-loss/

"70 Affirmations for Self-Worth and Love Yourself More." Posted by December 6, 2021. https://www.happierhuman.com/affirmations-self-worth/

Lebow, Hilary I., and Sandra Silva Casabianca. "Do You Know How to Manage Your Emotions and Why It Matters?" Posted April 6, 2022. https://psychcentral.com/health/emotional-regulation

Lee-Baggley, Dayna. "Why Self-Compassion Is Critical to Weight Management." Posted July 19, 2019. https://www.newharbinger. com/blog/self-help/why-self-compassion-is-critical-to-weight-management/

Live Well Dorset. "The Effects of Emotional Eating." Accessed November 11, 2022. https://www.livewelldorset.co.uk/articles/ the-effects-of-emotional-eating/

Marter, Joyce. "7 Ways to Ask for Emotional Support." Posted November 23, 2021. https://www.psychologytoday.com/us/blog/ mental-wealth/202111/7-ways-ask-emotional-support

Martin, Heather. "4 Negative Thoughts That Are Hindering Your Weight-Loss Goals—and How to Fix It." Posted June 29, 2022.

https://www.today.com/health/behavior/want-lose-weight-ditch-perfectionism-1-thing-instead-rcna35778

May, Michelle. "Emotional Eating." Accessed November 12, 2022. https://barriefht.ca/wp-content/uploads/2019/10/6.-Emotional-Eating.pdf

Mayo Clinic. "Hunger-Satiety Rating Scale." Accessed November 12, 2022. https://diabetes.org/sites/default/files/2019-06/hunger-rating-scale.pdf

"Weight Loss: Gain Control of Emotional Eating." Accessed November 11, 2022. https://www.mayoclinic.org/healthy-lifestyle/weight-loss/in-depth/weight-loss/art-20047342

McCallum, Katie. "A Dietitian's No-Nonsense Guide to Fighting Emotional Eating." Posted December 7, 2020. https://www.houston methodist.org/blog/articles/2020/dec/a-dietitians-no-nonsense-guide-to-fighting-emotional-eating/

McGonigal, Kelly. "The Problem with Dieting." Posted November 17, 2009. https://www.psychologytoday.com/us/blog/the-science-willpower/200911/the-problem-dieting

McQuillan, Susan. "8 Emotional Situations That Trigger Overeating." Posted September 6, 2019. https://www.psycom.net/emotions-that-trigger-overeating

Medline Plus. "Break the Bonds of Emotional Eating." Accessed November 12, 2022. https://medlineplus.gov/ency/patientinstruc tions/000808.htm

Mental Health America. "Helpful vs Harmful: Ways to Manage Emotions." Accessed November 12, 2022. https://www.mhana tional.org/helpful-vs-harmful-ways-manage-emotions

Mind Tools. "Cognitive Restructuring: Reducing Stress by Changing Your Thinking." Accessed November 12, 2022. https://www.mind tools.com/pages/article/newTCS_81.htm

Monge, Jessica. "Weight Loss: How to Stop Negative Self-Talk." Posted May 2021. https://www.lifeextension.com/wellness/weight/weight-loss-prevent-negative-self-talk

Motivation Weight Management. "10 Affirmations to Help with Your

Weight Loss Today!" Posted August 2, 2018. https://motivation.ie/
top-tips/positive-affirmations-help-weight-loss/

Nemours Children's Health. "Emotional Eating." Accessed November
12, 2022. https://kidshealth.org/en/teens/emotional-eating.html

Nutritious Life. "5 Common Types of Emotional Eaters." Accessed
November 11, 2022. https://nutriouslife.com/eat-empowered/
common-types-emotional-eaters/

Oliech, Mel and Ronnie. "How Low Self-Worth Affects Your Weight."
Accessed November 11, 2022. https://imanitribe.com/blog/how-
low-self-worth-affects-your-weight/

Oliveira, Rosane. "Emotions and Eating." Posted November 16, 2016.
https://pblife.org/health/emotions-and-eating/

Petre, Alina. "How to Meal Prep: A Beginner's Guide." Updated
September 30, 2018. https://www.healthline.com/nutrition/how-
to-meal-prep

Pezzolesi, Cinzia. "Emotional Eating: How We Try to Regulate Our
Emotions with Food and What We Should Do Instead." Accessed
November 12, 2022. https://insighttimer.com/blog/emotional-
eating-regulate-emotional-systems/

Plata, Mariana. "What You Might Need, Depending on How You're
Feeling." Posted March 28, 2020. https://www.psychologytoday.
com/us/blog/the-gen-y-psy/202003/what-you-might-need-
depending-how-youre-feeling

Positive Psychology Foundation, The. "How to Practice Self-Compassion, Lose Weight, and Feel Good about Yourself." Posted August
20, 2011. https://www.positivepsyc.com/blog/how-to-practice-
self-compassion-lose-weight-and-feel-good-about-yourself

Potter, Diana. "What Is Emotional Eating? My Story." Accessed
November 12, 2022. https://www.webmd.com/diet/obesity/
features/what-is-emotional-eating-my-story

Psychologies. "Test: Are You an Emotional Eater?" Posted February 12,
2016. https://www.psychologies.co.uk/test/test-are-you-an-
emotional-eater/

Psychology Compass. "5 Scientific Steps to Raise Your Emotional

Awareness and Gain Control." Accessed November 12, 2022. https://psychologycompass.com/blog/emotional-awareness/

Raypole, Crystal. "How to Identify and Manage Your Emotional Triggers." Posted November 13, 2020. https://www.healthline.com/health/mental-health/emotional-triggers

Richo, David. "13 Strategies to Deal with Your Emotional Triggers." Posted September 30, 2020. https://experiencelife.lifetime.life/article/13-strategies-to-deal-with-your-emotional-triggers/

Rittenhouse, Margot. "Overcoming Messages That Your Worth Is Based on Your Weight." Posted July 23, 2020. https://www.eatingdisorderhope.com/blog/overcoming-messages-self-worth-based-your-weight

Rose, Darya. "The Problem(s) with Dieting." Posted May 2, 2016. https://blog.myfitnesspal.com/the-problems-with-dieting/

Savage, Eliza. "1-Week Healthy and Balanced Meal Plan Ideas: Recipes and Prep." Updated August 24, 2022. https://www.verywellfit.com/an-example-of-a-healthy-balanced-meal-plan-2506647

Say, Nicholas. "6 Ways to Use Affirmations Effectively to Change Your Life." Posted March 24, 2020. https://www.happierhuman.com/use-affirmations/

Sisson, Mark. "Do You Use Food as a Crutch?" Posted December 12, 2013. https://www.marksdailyapple.com/do-you-use-food-as-a-crutch/

Smoke Free. "Set Healthy Eating Goals." Accessed November 12, 2022. https://smokefree.gov/stay-smokefree-good/eat-healthy/set-healthy-eating-goals

Stanborough, Rebecca Joy. "How to Change Negative Thinking with Cognitive Restructuring." Posted February 4, 2020. https://www.healthline.com/health/cognitive-restructuring

Streit, Lizzie. "SMART Goals for Healthy Eating and Weight Loss." Accessed November 12, 2022. https://www.healthyforlifemeals.com/blog/smart-goals-for-healthy-eating-and-weight-loss

Suazo, Amanda. "How to Meal Prep: A Beginner's Guide for Perfect Make-Ahead Meals." Accessed November 12, 2022. https://www.

bulletproof.com/diet/healthy-eating/how-to-meal-prep-begin ners-guide/

Tartakovsky, Margarita. "When Your Self-Worth Is Wrapped Around Your Weight (and 7 Ways to Unwrap It)." Posted January 14, 2010. https:// psychcentral.com/blog/weightless/2010/01/when-your-self-worth-is-wrapped-around-your-weight-and-7-ways-to-unwrap-it#1

Teich, Jessica. "The Unbearable Weight of Diet Culture." Updated January 29, 2021. https://www.goodhousekeeping.com/health/ diet-nutrition/a35036808/what-is-diet-culture/

University of New Hampshire. "Recognizing Emotions." Accessed November 12, 2022. https://www.unh.edu/pacs/recognizing-emotions

Unlock Food. "10 'SMART' Healthy Eating Goals." Accessed November 12, 2022. https://www.unlockfood.ca/en/Articles/Weight-and-Health/10-SMART%E2%80%9D-Healthy-Eating-Goals.aspx

Van Edwards, Vanessa. "Why Do We Eat? 10 Amazing Science Facts behind Our Eating Habits." Accessed November 12, 2022. https:// www.scienceofpeople.com/why-we-eat/

WebMD. "Emotional Eating: Feeding Your Feelings." Accessed November 12, 2022. https://www.webmd.com/diet/features/ emotional-eating-feeding-feelings

Weight Matters. "10 Ways to Manage Binge Eating Triggers." Accessed November 12, 2022. https://weightmatters.co.uk/2019/07/30/10-ways-manage-binge-eating-triggers/

Werner, Carly, and Aline Dias. "Emotional Eating: What You Should Know." Updated September 14, 2022. https://www.healthline.com/ health/emotional-eating

Whitehead, Erin. "10 Reasons You Eat When You're Not Actually Hungry." Posted August 9, 2011. https://www.sparkpeople.com/ resource/nutrition_articles.asp?id=1660

Willard, Christopher. "6 Ways to Practice Mindful Eating." Posted January 17, 2019. https://www.mindful.org/6-ways-practice-mind ful-eating/

Yes Health. "How to Know When You're Full." Posted September 27,

2018. https://blog.yeshealth.com/consumer/how-to-know-when-youre-full

Zelman, Kathleen M. "Why We Eat the Foods We Do." Accessed November 11, 2022. https://www.webmd.com/diet/features/why-we-eat-the-foods-we-do

Printed in Great Britain
by Amazon

21083953R00108